NHS plc

The Privatisation of
Our Health Care

◆

ALLYSON M. POLLOCK

with
COLIN LEYS, DAVID PRICE, DAVID ROWLAND
and SHAMINI GNANI

VERSO

London • New York

First published by Verso 2004

1 3 5 7 9 10 8 6 4 2

Verso
UK: 6 Meard Street, London W1F 0EG
USA: 180 Varick Street, New York, NY 10014−4606
www.versobooks.com

Verso is the imprint of New Left Books

ISBN 1−84467−011−2

British Library Cataloguing in Publication Data
Pollock, Allyson
  NHS plc: the privatisation of our health care
1. Great Britain. National Health Service 2. National health services −
Great Britain 3. Privatization − Great Britain
I. Title II. Leys, Colin, 1931−
362.1'0941

ISBN 1844670112

Library of Congress Cataloging-in-Publication Data
Pollock, Allyson.
  NHS plc: the privatisation of our health care / Allyson M. Pollock,
  with Colin Leys ... [et al.].
    p. ; cm.
      Includes bibliographical references and index.
      ISBN 1-84467-011-2 (hardcover : alk. paper)
1. Great Britain. National Health Service. 2. National health services −
Economic aspects − Great Britain. 3. Health services administration −
Great Britain. 4. Medical care − Great Britain − Finance. 5. Medical
policy − Great Britain. 6. Privatization − Great Britain.
[DNLM: 1. Great Britain. National Health Service. 2. State Medicine −
economics − Great Britain. 3. Health Care Sector − trends − Great
Britain. 4. Marketing of Health Services − economics − Great Britain.
5. Privatization − economics − Great Britain. W 225 FA1 P776n 2004]
I. Leys, Colin. II. Title.
RA412.5.G7P656 2004
362.1'0941--dc22

2004012869

Typeset in Bembo
Printed and bound in the UK by The Bath Press

CONTENTS

PREFACE

NHS plc is an account of how Britain's National Health Service, which established health care as a right, has been progressively dismantled and privatised by successive governments over the past quarter-century. The story is of course not unique to Britain. Universal health care systems are being dismantled and privatised across the world. Making health care once again a commodity to be bought, rather than a right, has become the standard prescription of the World Bank, the International Monetary Fund, the World Trade Organisation, and even the World Health Organisation – and, increasingly, the European Commission.

This book tries to show what is at stake. The dismantling process and its consequences are profoundly anti-democratic and opaque. The catchphrases of 'public–private partnerships', 'modernisation', 'value for money', 'local ownership' and the rest conceal the extent and real nature of what is happening; moreover, the complexity of health care allows the reality of its transformation into a market to be buried under a thousand half-truths. Some of the key turning points are briefly highlighted by some of the media, but the systematic nature of the process is hidden in the rhetoric of 'diversity' and 'choice'.

NHS plc aims to record what has been happening in an accurate and accessible way. The public have a right to know, even if the process has already gone too far to be easily or quickly reversed. The book begins by showing the commercial forces at work in the accelerating privatisation process, and what the real costs of privatisation are – both the dramatically increased financial costs of using private enterprise, which is in reality so much *less* efficient in providing health care, and the costs in terms of lost services, lost universality and lost equality. It offers a summary of the overall process and then describes what this means in each of three core sectors of health care: hospitals, primary care and long-term care for older people. Finally it records some of the ways in which the process has been pushed ahead at the expense of truth and objectivity in public policy-making – how scientific evidence has been ignored, distorted and even invented, and objective criticism has been suppressed.

Although the book draws on twenty years' experience of day-to-day work in the NHS and research projects related to it, and the contributions of many colleagues in diverse disciplines, it does not pretend to offer anything like a complete picture. The consequences of political devolution in Wales and Scotland are not covered. For more than fifty years the UK NHS has been the model maker for universal health care, its systems designed and copied throughout the world. However, as it turns to embrace market forces and in the process exports the new model worldwide, it is important to understand that not all parts of the UK are following suit. While England is fast becoming the laboratory and test bed for market-driven experiments, Scotland and Wales are currently trying to minimise the effects of the market forces that were unleashed throughout the 1990s – and with some success. Although the Treasury and Westminster have thrust upon Scotland and Wales the pernicious policy of public–private partnerships and private finance, both countries have begun to take small steps to undo the internal market, trying to strengthen public health functions and restore some basic planning functions. They have eschewed foundation trusts, resisted expanding the private sector and withstood the drive to implement the complex US-derived pricing system upon which a market depends. But the pressure on politicians to take England's route is intense and should not be underestimated. Every policy failure is seized upon as a justification for abandoning the NHS and turning to markets. I hope this book may help give policy-makers and politicians the courage to stick to the principles that guided their predecessors in establishing universal health care.

Important issues such as services for people with mental illnesses, learning disabilities or physical disabilities, for example, are also not covered in this book. Neither are key services such as pathology, radiology and other diagnostic services, and paramedical services such as chiropody, physiotherapy, dietetics and speech therapy. Another major story omitted here is the erosion of all public health functions and the retreat of public health from service planning. The assessment of health care needs and service planning has become a lost discipline, and the information systems and data collection that would allow the monitoring of the decay and growing inequities are being destroyed. What would the great champions of public health like William Farr, Edwin Chadwick, Florence Nightingale and William Henry Duncan make of the wanton destruction of our public institutions and systems of public accountability? For the policy prescriptions being applied to hospitals, primary care and long-term care are being applied to all these fields too, with equally costly and unfair consequences.

It also needs acknowledging that the people on whom all the NHS's services depend – its nurses, paramedics, pharmacists, physiotherapists, administrators, porters, cleaners, laboratory and other technical workers, to mention only a few – are also omitted from this account. Another book would be needed to do justice to their contributions, and the way privatisation has affected them. Many feel increasingly disenfranchised, under-supported and under-resourced, and no longer able to provide, let alone develop, services they know patients need. Service innovation and innovative research have also become difficult without financial backing from commercial sources, and the focus on league tables and 'superstars' means that quiet, low-cost but 'unprofitable' innovations, and the people who make them, too often go unnoticed. Some despair and consider leaving for the private sector. This book should help to explain why the systems they now find themselves working in are becoming increasingly alienating, and show why and how commercial values are increasingly displacing the service ethos in which they were trained. It may also help them to see that other solutions are possible and that the market model is not the only alternative.

For this book is above all an expression of hope for the future. One day people will demand the restoration of a national health service, but the institutional memory will have been lost. Clear accounts of what its guiding principles were, and the structures, organisations and funding mechanisms needed to achieve them, will be at a premium. So too will an account of its weaknesses and problems – the better to design them out in the future. The market paradigm is rapidly becoming the only one we know. But the universal health care paradigm requires a different approach. It needs mechanisms that enable cross-subsidisation and risk-pooling between rich and poor, healthy and sick, town and country. But these protective mechanisms are being abandoned, and collectivism and compassion are being replaced by individualism (in reality 'choice' means that patients learn to believe that with sufficient information they can access better health care than others) and hard-nosed business tactics. 'Targeting' services to serve the greatest needs sounds fair but actually means the loss of both preventive and integrated health care, as well as the holistic approach, and a return to what Richard Titmuss rightly called 'residual' forms of welfare.

The era in which the judge and the janitor would have beds on the same ward, and receive the same standard of care, is drawing to a close. Professionals who worked to build up services to give the best possible quality of care to all patients are being replaced with agents acting on behalf of corporations and their shareholders. The requirement laid on foundation trusts to generate surpluses means that care will increasingly be oriented to the more profitable treatments, and to patients who can afford to pay. Meanwhile the health service is being broken up into hundreds of competing trading organisations. Inevitably some will go to the wall and there will be more closures and mergers. Health care will revert towards the pre-NHS situation, with a lucky few having access to superior care while most of the population makes do with increasingly limited 'basic' services of declining quality.

It took more than fifty years to build the consensus for the NHS, and it is a testimony to what can be achieved with the right sort of political will. It is hoped that this book will help inspire a new generation to work towards reclaiming the rights and entitlements that the NHS once conferred, and a new vision of health care for all.

ACKNOWLEDGEMENTS

This book reflects the spirit and work of the Public Health Policy Unit at University College London. It has been a team effort. Colin Leys guided the project, believed in it and kept it going against all the odds. In a small unit with slender resources and competing pressures this has been no easy task. He was responsible for helping me shape the book, reading and editing all its contents, and drafting the political account in Chapter 3. David Price was responsible for researching and initially drafting Chapter 4, on acute hospitals, while Chapter 6, on long-term care, was researched and drafted by David Rowland; Chapter 5, on primary care, was researched and drafted by Shamini Gnani. We discussed and commented on all the drafts together.

Every chapter in *NHS plc* draws heavily on contributions by and collaborations with others, although I take full responsibility for any errors in the analysis or shortcomings in the evidence it may contain. It is not possible here to name all those who helped but some people deserve special mention. Neil Vickers, Sylvia Godden, Jean Shaoul, Matthew Dunnigan, Declan Gaffney, Alison Talbot-Smith, Alison Macfarlane, Sue Kerrison, Stewart Player, Naomi Pfeffer, Michel Coleman, Margaret Whitehead, Karin Janzon, Stella Law, Rosalind Raine, Charlene Harrington, John Mohan, Azeem Majeed and James Lancaster have all collaborated on aspects of the research which has been central to the unit's work and which underpins this book. Their contributions have been invaluable, as has James Lancaster's tireless support.

The book has also been inspired by the contributions of many others, including members of the public, campaign groups and public health academics actively seeking to defend the public's rights and entitlements to health care. Maria Goldenberg of the Bromley Community Care Protection Group, the hospital campaign groups at Swindon, Norfolk & Norwich, Birmingham and Calderdale deserve special mention, as do Richard Taylor MP and John Ball in Kidderminster, Lord Hattersley, Will Hutton, John Lister at London Health Emergency, the Radical Statistics Group, Ursula Pearce and the late Lord Howell in Birmingham, John Sewell, Peter Fisher and all the members of the NHS Consultants' Association, Harry Keen and the NHS Support Federation, Brian Potter, formerly of the Scottish BMA, Ron Singer and other members of the Medical Practitioners Union, Sir Iain Chalmers, Margaret Whitehead, Sir Denis Pereira Gray of the Nuffield Trust, Aileen Clarke, Ian Basnett, and Martin McKee of the European Observatory on Health Care Systems, all of whom continue to work tirelessly and selflessly to promote and defend universal access to health care. Malcolm Wing and Margie Jaffe at UNISON, together with Jon Ford and Sir Sandy Macara at the BMA, commissioned the unit's first report into the Private Finance Initiative, while Martin McIvor at Catalyst and John Edmonds at the GMB also gave us support. Steffie Woolhandler and all the Physicians for a National Health Program in the US, Pedro Marcet in Spain, and Hixinio Beiras and Marciano Sanchez Bayle of the Spanish Federation of Associations for the Defence of Public Health, Colleen and John Fuller and Verna Milligan at the Canadian Health Coalition, Alexis Benos and members of the International Association of Health Policy, Meri Koisovolo, Andy Wynne at the Association of Chartered Certified Accountants, Marc de Bruycker in Brussels, Richard Smith at the *British Medical Journal*, Richard Horton at the *Lancet*, and many others have all variously come to the unit's aid and helped us understand the international significance of this project.

Among the numerous public health colleagues who have lent their support to our work over the years across many different public health departments are Jane Jackson, Ross Anderson, Jean Richards, Hilary Stirland, Penny Bevan, Jacky Chambers, and Michael Marmot. Special thanks also go to Robert Naylor, David Fish, Richard Frackowiak, and the many other colleagues at University College London Hospitals and

University College London who have always taken great care to respect the unit's right to continue its academic work independent of my NHS commitments. Journalists Paul Foot, Nick Cohen, the late Arnold Kemp, Nick Mathiason, Felicity Lawrence, Seumas Milne, Anne McGauran, Melanie McFadyean, John Carvel, Brian Christie, and many others have ensured that the debate on entitlements and rights to health care is not extinguished. Special stalwarts of the NHS include Charles Webster, the former official historian of the NHS, who has given us a wonderful legacy of documentary evidence, Julian Tudor Hart, the late Sir Douglas Black, and Sir George Godber. They count among the true architects of the NHS and their example gave us the courage to continue when the going got rough. Last but not least there are the many friends and family members who have always been there when things were difficult and when political interference threatened to extinguish the unit. They debated the issues and put up the counter-arguments.

I hope that thanks to all these people's efforts readers of this book will be able to understand why universal health care and its organisation really matter.

LIST OF ACRONYMS

BMA	British Medical Association
CHAI	Commission for Healthcare Audit and Inspection (Healthcare Commission)
CHI	Commission for Health Improvement
DGH	district general hospital
DTC	Diagnostic and Treatment Centre
EU	European Union
FCE	finished consultant episode
GATS	General Agreement on Trade in Services
GDP	gross domestic product
GMS	general medical services
GP	general practitioner
GPFC	General Practice Finance Corporation
HCP	Health Care Projects
HMO	Health Maintenance Organisation
IFSL	International Financial Services London
IHA	Independent Healthcare Association
IPPR	Institute for Public Policy Research
ITC	independent treatment centre

LIFT	local improvement finance trust
NHS	National Health Service
NICE	National Institute for Clinical Excellence
OECD	Organisation for Economic Cooperation and Development
PCG	primary care group
PCT	primary care trust
PFI	Private Finance Initiative
PMS	Personal Medical Services
PPP	public–private partnership
PSS	Personal Social Services
PUK	Partnerships UK
RAWP	Resource Allocation Working Party
SHA	strategic health authority
SPV	special purpose vehicle
STG	Special Transition Grant
UCLH	University College London Hospitals NHS Trust
WTO	World Trade Organisation

I

MARKET PRESCRIPTIONS

Perhaps nothing sums up the state of the National Health Service today as well as the credentials of the people who are now at its helm. Its senior managers now include people with no training or experience in public health or the principles of health care delivery: arts graduates of all descriptions, ex-army officers, and, increasingly, people seeking a change from private enterprise (or surplus to its needs) – former choco-late and biscuit manufacturers, bank managers, chief executives of housing corporations. Many in this new management cadre are capable administrators but all of them – including those with substantial expe-rience in the service – are now obliged to conform to an essentially business culture. The main qualification for running the NHS now is knowledge of business methods – and, it sometimes seems, a P45 from industry or commerce, which also supply most of the non-executive members of hospital, health authority and primary care trust boards. Doctors, nurses, public health specialists and other health care profes-sionals do not feature except at the front line – a crass but intended result of politicians' preoccupation with quelling what they call the 'producer' interests of those delivering hands-on care.

The permeation of NHS management and hospital and health authority boards by business is emblematic of the way in which private enterprise is penetrating and corroding the fabric of the NHS at every level. The NHS, with its enormous range of activities and £74 billion annual turnover, offers marvellous opportunities for companies seeking security of income and healthy profits. Health care corporations, pharmaceutical companies and the construction industry are finding lucrative new openings in the NHS, thanks to Labour's strategy of privatisation and public–private partnerships.

In pole position is the transnational pharmaceutical industry, which currently takes an estimated 14 per cent of NHS expenditure – more than £10 billion a year. Closely following is the construction industry, in collaboration with bankers, venture capitalists and service operators. Companies like Balfour Beatty, Tarmac, Jarvis and Siemens are reaping the rewards of multimillion-pound Private Finance Initiative (PFI) hospital contracts, under which these hospitals are committed to handing over 12 to 20 per cent of their annual income for thirty years or more. On the fringes are a myriad of advisers and subcontractors vying for contracts for supplying anything from information technology and building and equipment maintenance to human resources and agency nursing staff. The grand London offices of large legal and accounting firms such as Herbert Smith, Eversheds, PricewaterhouseCoopers and KPMG are now furnished to a significant extent from fees paid out of NHS funds: funds that would once have paid for long-term care, or speech therapy for people with strokes, or chiropody for millions of older people and people with diabetes – NHS services that have become increasingly rare to their grateful recipients. And now also pressing forward to centre stage are the big national and increasingly transnational health care corporations such as BUPA, PPP, United HealthCare, Kaiser Permanente, Westminster Health Care and Capio, seeking new market opportunities through joint ventures with the NHS.

No one knows quite how much NHS money is being diverted out of clinical care and into the pockets of the private sector, because the public expenditure data do not reveal it, and neither do NHS accounts. The public are constantly being told about all the money going into the NHS, but not about how their taxes are propping up and cosseting companies whose profitability and stockmarket positions frequently depend entirely on their intimate relationships with the NHS.[1]

In the early days of power the new Labour government was on a charm offensive and wanted to be seen to be listening, and so Geoffrey Robinson, a former businessman and now Paymaster-General, agreed to meet me in his office at the foot of Downing Street to discuss Labour's embrace of the PFI, whereby the government contracts with the private sector to borrow money on its behalf. The ceiling of his vast office was covered in heavy ornate plasterwork and hung with chandeliers. An enormous carved mahogany desk, the only sign that this was an office, was dwarfed by drawing-room furniture, a handsome rug and some richly upholstered couches on which we sat. He listened politely to my analysis of the PFI, based on a detailed study of PFI business cases, his chief aide taking copious notes while we drank tea. When I was done, Robinson responded by praising the virtues of the private sector and inviting me to join him for a drink on the terrace of the House of Commons.

An even more significant figure who did not care to engage in a serious discussion of the issues was the Chancellor of the Exchequer, Gordon Brown. In 2002 I asked him if he could explain the rationale behind the use of private finance for public investment, given that private borrowing was more expensive, and the risks were not in practice transferred to the private sector. His response was simply to declare repeatedly that the public sector is bad at management, and that only the private sector is efficient and can manage services well. By 2003 the business paradigm was the only model that Treasury and senior Department of Health officials could relate to.

New Labour's penchant for appointing large numbers of young, mainly male policy advisers in Numbers 10 and 11 Downing Street, and the inner offices of cabinet ministers, was a preference not just for youth, but also for receptiveness to market ideology. Soon these inner sanctums – modern baronial courts – were full of people drawn from policy think-thanks such as the IPPR, Demos and the Social Market Foundation, heavily sponsored by and networked into industry. They came primed with the doctrines of 'the new public management', courtesy of the US Commonwealth Fund scholarships and business or public administration courses at Harvard. Simon Stevens, Robert Hill, Geoff Mulgan, Andrew Adonis and the Miliband brothers and others were swiftly promoted to be senior policy aides to Blair and Brown. Some later became MPs, others corporate executives and advisers.

THE REVOLVING DOOR BETWEEN THE NHS AND BUSINESS

The incoming Labour government also imported a cohort of mainly young people from the private sector to be civil servants on secondment, thereby opening what rapidly became a great revolving door between the public and private spheres. Briefly heading the PFI unit in the NHS, for example, was Robert Osborne, on secondment from the construction company Tarmac, a major beneficiary of PFI (later 'public–private partnership' or PPP) contracts. Richard Granger, a 37-year-old former management consultant to Deloitte & Touche, was appointed director-general of NHS information technology at £250,000 a year – around £90,000 more than the NHS chief executive, Nigel Crisp, received. The new government also lifted the ban that had been imposed on further government contracts with the auditing firm Arthur Andersen – for having, in the previous government's view, failed to advise the government adequately – and in 1998 appointed as Economic Secretary to the Treasury the new MP Patricia Hewitt, a former director of research for Arthur Andersen Consulting (Arthur Andersen's management consultancy arm). Several lucrative PFI contracts with the firm followed.[2]

Another key figure in the commercialisation of the public service was Dame Sheila Masters (later Baroness Noakes) from KPMG, another large management consultant firm. During an earlier secondment to the Treasury she had been instrumental in persuading the Conservative government to abandon the Ryrie rules – rules that protected public sector expenditure from the inroads of venture capitalists and bankers. Now she was brought back to advise Gordon Brown and the Department of Health. Under the Conservatives her market prescriptions for the public sector had included 'resource accounting', which was to play a special role in the break-up of the NHS, and helped to establish the accounting rules for the NHS 'internal market' and other public services. Labour put her in charge of a review of the NHS 'estate' – its land and buildings – making her a key player in the ensuing great sell-off of NHS property. Her report, *Sold on Health*, had extensive input from private sector property owners, developers and agents, as well as public sector organisations with large property portfolios. It aimed 'to root out surplus estate, accelerate sales and cut red tape'.[3] Among many other key positions, in 2000 she was also President of the Institute of Chartered Accountants and played a role in determining the rules governing where PFI contracts figured in the government's accounts.

Also from KPMG came Tim Stone, who advised on the PFI policy and then became involved in selling public–private partnerships abroad through International Financial Services London (IFSL), which represents the UK services industry on the UK Government's Trade Policy Consultative Forum for the WTO negotiations on the Geneal Agreement on Trade in Services (GATS). IFSL organises meetings and programmes for overseas officials visiting London from countries as diverse as Germany and Egypt, Canada and Mexico, who come to find out more about the UK's experience and expertise in PFI/PPP.

Before Labour came to power in 1997 I had been invited by a friend to discuss PFI over lunch with a merchant banker who was responsible for the development of project finance for financing public services at BZW. We ate in the bank's private dining room with a prime view over the Thames. Black-coated waiters, who seemed to outnumber us by about two to one, served a lunch that lasted almost three hours. When I wryly observed that he might like to try our hospital canteen at St George's Hospital in south London, he laughed heartily. He explained how using the PFI would 'take the fat' out of the NHS and introduce new efficiencies, and enthused about the savings to be made from cutting the number of hospital support staff. I could not help thinking of the rows of terraced houses in the impoverished community of Tooting from which St George's mainly female, mainly black ancillary workforce is drawn.

It was not long before the merchant bankers were moving across to take key posts in the public sector. Adrian Montague, a corporate lawyer and co-head of Global Project Finance at the merchant bank Dresdner Kleinwort Benson was a prime example.

Within months of Labour's coming to power Montague had become the £160,000-a-year head of Gordon Brown's Treasury taskforce on PFI, Partnerships UK (PUK), responsible for drawing up the rules for handing over the future of hospitals and schools to banks and construction firms. His PUK role was in addition to his one-day-a-week, £30,000-a-year job as Private Finance Adviser to the Minister of Transport on the privatisation of London Underground – and yet another as adviser to the giant French bank, Société Générale, the largest shareholder in Alcatel, one of the firms bidding to privatise the Underground. He had played a pivotal role in drawing up the contracts for electricity privatisation. Within months of Montague's appointment to the Treasury taskforce the first PFI contracts were being signed and ancillary hospital staff were being transferred to the private sector, with the subsequent erosion of rights for all new employees. In 2003 Montague left PUK to become, in effect, an overseas ambassador for the policy, selling the UK model of PPPs abroad for the management consultancy World Wide Business Research, promoting expensive conferences and trading on his experience and connections as a former adviser to the Treasury and the Department of Transport.

At the same time, faced with the escalating costs of privatisation, Gordon Brown asked Derek Wanless, the former head of NatWest Bank, to report to him on the future funding of the NHS. The terms of reference of the report were restricted to issues of funding, not service delivery. Wanless's final report, in 2002, *Securing Our Future Health*, recommended both the continuation of tax-based funding as the fairest and least expensive way of redistributing resources, and a major injection of new funding, which Blair and his government endorsed.[4] No mention was made of where much of that new money would go. The private healthcare sector, however, was given a strong signal that this commitment meant that investments in health care provision would be repaid out of future tax revenues.

It was clear that the Secretary of State for Health at the time, Alan Milburn, fully endorsed this message. In office from 1999 to 2003 he ardently promoted the use of private finance and negotiated a so-called Concordat with the private sector that explicitly invited it to start bidding to take over NHS clinical services. And when he left office Milburn himself used the revolving door, becoming a £30,000-a-year adviser to Bridgepoint, a venture capital firm heavily involved in financing private health care firms moving into the NHS. Bridgepoint's interests include Alliance Medical, a private operator of diagnostic imaging equipment; Match Group, a health care staffing agency; Medica, a nursing homes operator; and Robina Care Group, a provider of specialist residential care.[5]

BLURRED BOUNDARIES

Given the new management culture it probably should not have been a cause for surprise that businessmen appointed to the boards of hospital trusts, and some senior managers of trusts, were soon selling their inside knowledge of the NHS to the private sector. A good example came to light in 2001 when the planned £600 million rebuilding of St Bartholomew's Hospital in London was referred to the government amid allegations of a conflict of interest. The local patients' watchdog, the City and Hackney Community Health Council, accused one of the two companies bidding for the lucrative contract, Skanska/Innisfree, of possessing 'immense inner knowledge'. Skanska/Innisfree's bid was being handled by Health Care Projects (HCP), which stood to make around £350,000 a year in management fees if Skanska/Innisfree was successful.[6] HCP had been founded by Gerry Green, who until 1997 was chief executive at Bart's (as St Bartholomew's Hospital is commonly called) and who, according to HCP's own website, while employed by the NHS 'led the proposal to develop the Royal London Hospital, the most extensive hospital scheme in the PFI programme'.[7] In 2003 HCP employed six former directors of the Bart's and Royal London Hospitals Trust including Ray Pett, who until 2000 was the trust's chief executive; Peter Holden, its former director of facilities; and Barry Clarke, the current deputy director of facilities, both of whom worked as HCP consultants while still employed by the trust. Jackie Cardiff, who until January 2001 was the trust's director of operations, was also an HCP employee in 2003, and Sir Derek Boorman, the trust's chairman from 1994 to 1997, was an HCP director. In November 2003 the government signed a contract for the rebuild, awarding the biggest PFI hospital contract yet, worth in excess of £1 billion, to Skanska/Innisfree.

Another example of the increasingly blurred public–private boundary is the role of Dr Chai Patel. Chai Patel acquired Priory Healthcare, which had been founded by an American company based in California, and in 2000 merged it with the Specialist Healthcare Services Division of his former company, Westminster Health Care, to create the Priory Group. As chief executive of Westminster Health Care he had been paid £443,000 a year, making him one of the highest-paid health-care chief executives in the UK. His acquisition of the Priory Group and the sale of Westminster Health Care increased his wealth by an estimated £8 million.[8] The millionaire doctor-turned-businessman advised the prime minister's office on private sector involvement in the NHS, and was a member of the Department of Health's taskforce for older people and better regulation, until forced to step down as a government adviser on the elderly (as well as from the board of Help the Aged) following a devastating report into one of Westminster Health Care's nursing homes (see Chapter 6). By the mid-1990s, however, Westminster Health Care, in addition to providing care home services for older people, had diversified into specialist mental health and related areas such as acute psychiatric hospitals, brain injury centres, addiction centres and secure mental health services. Patel's new company, the Priory Group, acquired these assets and added them to its existing portfolio, which included special education facilities, including residential special schools, for young people with emotional and behavioural difficulties, mild learning difficulties, autism and Asperger's syndrome.[9] By 2003 it owned sixteen psychiatric hospitals, four special schools, two therapeutic community assessment services, five brain injury/rehabilitation units and four secure and step-down units, and was in a powerful position to lobby for more government contracts and NHS funding, having largely cornered this market.

A case particularly heavy with future significance was that of Bill Moyes, the director of strategic planning and performance management of the management executive of NHS Scotland from 1990 to 1994, and a key adviser on Edinburgh Infirmary's PFI project. Moyes left to join the Bank of Scotland Group, where he became head of infrastructure investment and set up the group's Private Finance Initiative team, which was involved in £500 million worth of NHS and education PFI schemes over six years.[10] He then moved on in July 2000 to become director-general of the British Retail Consortium, and after this spell in commerce was appointed by the Secretary of State in late 2003 to be the first independent regulator of the NHS – with huge powers, as we shall see, to determine the shape and culture of the NHS in the years to come.

By the middle of Labour's second term, public–private partnerships permeated every layer of the public sector. Concerned NHS staff (such as the BMA and the NHS Consultants' Association) or anyone else who saw career patterns such as the ones mentioned here as involving conflicts of interest were increasingly dismissed as naïve or self-interested. Public servants who were unwilling or unable to go along with the trend had by then largely been squeezed out through retirement, restructuring and retrenchment. By the late 1990s medical and nursing professionals were given senior posts only if they demonstrated a willingness to work with the private sector and put 'new public management' techniques into practice. In 2003, for instance, the Labour government appointed 'Czars' for every major disease specialty. Their key qualification was a willingness to implement the market revolution and inspire the rank and file to follow it. The first 'drug Czar', Keith Hellawell, refused to go along with New Labour's cavalier attitude to evidence-based policy-making, opposing the reclassification of cannabis, and was promptly sidelined.[11] At the same time the Department of Health was being remodelled, with a Department of Capacity and Choice replacing service planning. There was also a new section to promote the 'independent sector', and in particular the government's latest instant fix of 'surgical factories': privately run Diagnostic and Treatment Centres or DTCs. The idea was that the private sector would be encouraged to take on low-risk, high-turnover patients for elective procedures such as cataract surgery and hip replacements, in return for bringing in private finance and injecting new capacity – a fundamentally flawed idea, as we will see in Chapter 3.

THE INCOMING GLOBAL HEALTH CARE INDUSTRY

The new market supremos appointed to run the NHS would play a powerful role in promoting and serving the interests of business, attacking the service from within and without, and shaping its policies and structures to meet the needs of their commercial colleagues. With business patronage they were well equipped to do so. The government had begun by privatising non-clinical services and infrastructure. Now it began to extend the remit of the private sector from infrastructure projects to clinical care. In 2003 the government appointed a Texan, Ken Anderson, from the British facilities management company AMEY, to direct the programme promoting the new privately owned DTCs.[12] AMEY ran into serious financial difficulties over its accounting treatment of the PFI facilities it was providing to government, for failing to declare its bidding costs on the profit-and-loss account. But AMEY was just one of many UK companies that had cut their teeth on NHS infrastructure and facilities management contracts. Now, with the prospect of the privatisation of NHS clinical services, UK PFI consortia started teaming up with larger, multinational health care corporations to compete for the NHS funds that would flow to the providers of these services, repackaging themselves in a variety of new consortia.

Patients Choice Partners, for example, is a consortium that includes Nestor Healthcare, 'the UK's leading independent provider of personnel and service solutions to the health and social care market'; Carillion, a major UK construction and facilties management company with large hospital PFI contracts in the UK and Canada; and the South African private hospital group Medi-clinic.[13] Mercury Health Ltd., a subsidiary of Tribal Group plc, which claims to work with 90 per cent of the strategic health authorities and 75 per cent of NHS trusts, provides consultancy and professional support services to the public and private sectors in the UK, employing 1,200 people in forty-five offices. Mercury heads a consortium that includes Ascent Health (formerly Johnson & Johnson pharmaceuticals), Sanare, Reed Health Group, Match Group, Deluca Medical, and Parsons and Tyco. SECTA – another part of Tribal Group – was awarded the first franchise to take over the management of a 'failing' NHS hospital, the Good Hope Hospital in Birmingham, in 2002.

Examples of consortia involving UK and foreign companies include InterHealth Jarvis, which combines InterHealth Canada, a Canadian company that 'operates hospitals and other healthcare facilities in partnership with public and academic organisations' in Canada, with Jarvis, a leading UK facilities management and construction company that has some of the major PFI contracts for the public sector, including hospitals such as University College London Hospitals. Another consortium combines New York Presbyterian Healthcare System, which operates the New York Presbyterian Hospital, with WS Atkins, a leading UK facilities management and support service company.

Private health care providers in the UK were also among the bidders for the NHS waiting list elective work. They included BMI Healthcare, 'the UK's leading provider of independent healthcare, with nearly 50 hospitals nation-wide'; BUPA Hospitals Division, an independent health care insurer and provider which runs a number of hospitals in the UK and also has an international division; Capio Healthcare, a Swedish-based company but already one of the UK's leading independent providers of hospital services, with twenty-one acute units throughout the country; Nuffield Hospitals, 'a leading UK independent healthcare group with over 40 independent and charitable units operating nation-wide'; and Boots, the high-street chemist, which had already begun to branch out from providing NHS eye tests to doing eye surgery, offering laser treatment largely unavailable on the NHS, and then expanding into cataract surgery. But the for-profit domestic sector found it difficult to compete with inter-national companies, as foreign governments lost no time in promoting their own companies, all eager to take a slice of UK tax revenues.

In 2003, as part of the dissolution of the NHS into a 'mixed economy of health care', the Department of Health website published a shortlist of companies that were bidding to provide rapid diagnostic and treat-ment services to the NHS. These services had a special appeal to the private sector: they were low-risk, high-profit business opportunities, based on careful risk selection and low-risk medical procedures. Among the first off the starting block was Anglo-Canadian Clinics – an Alberta-based consortium that includes Calgary Health Region, the University of Calgary Medical Group, Surgical Centres Inc., Accommodata Ltd., Bowmer & Kirkland Ltd., Yorkon Ltd., and Torex Medical Systems Ltd. In Canada, for-profit health care is in effect prohibited under the Canada Health Act, and Canadians were concerned that this commer-cial foray was a sign of things to come for them.[14] Then from South Africa there was Care UK Afrox, a partnership between Care UK, which operates nursing and residential homes in the UK, and African Oxygen Ltd, a medical gases company that is part of BOC's medical group.

Another bidder was Netcare, the largest integrated private health care organisation in South Africa, which owns and manages 45 hospitals comprising 7,200 beds, 319 operating theatres and 61 specialised medical centres – in a country whose health care system mirrors that of the US in its extreme inequality between rich and poor. Netcare will be operating within a consortium that includes UK-based facilities management and construction companies. In September 2003 it signed its fourth contract with the NHS, to provide orthopaedic procedures for the NHS in Portsmouth, and was named the likely preferred bidder for two new fast-track treatment centres in the UK. An article in a South African business newspaper reported 'that the deal will strengthen Netcare's foothold in the UK, as well as boost its foreign earnings potential, while helping retain South African medical staff'.[15] However Netcare's forays into the UK health care arena caused controversy when a contract to provide NHS cataract operations to patients in Morecambe left 3 patients out of the 900 treated with a serious and rare infection – endophthalmitis – causing one to lose an eye. The contract between Netcare and Morecambe NHS Trust was referred to the Commission for Healthcare Audit and Inspection.[16]

From Germany came DTC International, a consortium including the German Medicine Network and Costain Construction. And from the USA came Healthmark Partners, which 'owns and operates specialty surgical facilities, both inpatient and outpatient, in joint ventures' with local physicians in the USA.[17] This, however, was a relatively minor player on the US health care scene, whose major players, backed by the most powerful state in the world, were bound to play a leading and influential role in the new British 'mixed economy of health care'.

And here we encounter a significant fact: by the time they began targeting UK public funds some US health care firms had changed their names, apparently in the hope of shedding images tarnished by a history of malfeasance and fraud in the USA. Among the leading bidders, for instance, was HCA Healthcare, which owns and operates around 200 hospitals and health care facilities in the USA, the UK and Switzerland. As Columbia/HCA it is the largest for-profit health care corporation in the USA. In December 2000 Columbia/HCA pleaded guilty to substantial criminal conduct and paid out $840 million in criminal fines and penalties; by June 2003, when the action by the US Department of Justice was finally settled, HCA had been required to pay out $1.7 billion for defrauding the US government and paying kickbacks to physicians, the largest case of health fraud in US history.* Now

---

* The US government also joined a suit against KPMG, the accounting firm which had allegedly helped Columbia/HCA to defraud the government, and recovered $9 million in fines and penalties in October 2001.

Columbia calls itself just HCA, since the old name has become synony-
mous 'with an aggressive culture'.[18] Another candidate currently
providing residential care in the UK is the US company Tenet. Tenet
used to be National Medical Enterprises, which paid $379 million to
the federal government in 1994 to settle what was then the largest-ever
US case of health care fraud.[19]

These cases are notorious, but not unique. Health care fraud is
endemic in the US system.[20] But this did not deter the Secretary of
State for Health, Alan Milburn, from announcing in October 2002, after
talks with the US Health Secretary, Tommy Thompson, that he was
signing a major contract with United HealthCare for advice on how to
cut costs in the NHS by keeping elderly patients out of hospital – a
scheme known as Evercare. The company was hired initially to help
design, monitor and advise on the running of ten pilot schemes in north,
south and west Bristol, Dorset, South Gloucestershire and Yorkshire.
Perhaps Milburn took heart from the fact that United HealthCare had
agreed to pay only some $7 million in fines in the previous two years,
after being charged with cheating the US government, doctors and
patients.[21]

The company paid $2.9 million in November 2002 to settle claims
that it had charged the US government for care to patients who it falsely
claimed were in nursing homes. In July 2002, moreover, the New York
State Insurance Department fined United HealthCare $1.5 million for
'cheating patients out of money': when patients were denied health care
payments under their insurance programme, some were given wrong
information by the company on how to appeal against this. Since March
2000 United HealthCare has also paid out almost $2 million in penalties
in nine different US states, including Florida, Texas, Ohio and New
Jersey, for a variety of different offences, including passing work to a
doctor whose medical licence had been revoked. The company's reputation was further damaged when vice-president Michael Mooney was
jailed for three and a half years in August 2002 and fined $220,000 for
insider trading.

The Evercare scheme has been publicly praised by President George
Bush – who with Dick Cheney received a personal 2004 campaign
contribution of $1.5 million from William W. McGuire, the CEO of
United HealthCare, making the latter a 'Bush–Cheney Pioneer' – but

academic research shows that it operates by restricting care to the patients it thinks it can make money out of.[22] When asked about the firm's catalogue of fines, a spokeswoman for the Department of Health told the *Observer* that this was part and parcel of operating in the health industry in the USA. She added: 'We are entirely satisfied that the procurement process was correctly followed before signing the deal.'[23] In May 2004 Blair's senior health policy adviser, Simon Stevens, and Richard Smith, the editor of the *British Medical Journal*, announced that they were leaving to join United HealthCare, now renamed the United Health Group, as the Group's Europe President and CEO, respectively.

SELLING OUT THE NHS

The effects of all this are more fundamental than solely a growth in opportunities for dubious business practices, or the diversion of tax revenues into the pockets of shareholders. What is occurring is an accelerating erosion, and increasingly a reversal, of what the NHS was created to achieve: making health care a right, and no longer something that could be bought or sold. When Aneurin Bevan, the NHS's key founder, spoke of freedom from fear, everyone understood what he meant. Before 1948, doctors had to decide whether a patient could afford to pay or should go without care. The distinguished GP Julian Tudor Hart tells a story of a colleague leaving behind a pair of gloves on the hallstand so that he could have an excuse to visit a sick child again without charging. With a National Health Service such gestures were to be replaced by an ethos according to which providing health services would be neither an opportunity to make money nor a charity. While financial contributions should be on the basis of ability to pay, there should be no link between service and payment in the mind of either the giver of the service or the recipient. Everyone should feel they had paid collectively for the service, through progressive taxation, and that it would be there when they needed it.

In practice, serious compromises were necessary in order to bring the NHS into being. The country was broke and Bevan was unable to persuade the Treasury, faced with the heavy cost of nationalising the hospitals, to buy out GP surgeries as well, and so GPs were allowed to remain self-employed small businesses, as were dentists, opticians and community pharmacists. Their status as 'independent contractors' to the NHS was a weakness which would be exploited by proponents of the market over the following decades. And while hospitals were nationalised, community health services, preventative services, child health, public health, and ambulance services remained the responsibility of local government, though funded by the NHS. This eventually led to a distinction between health care, which was free, and 'personal' or 'social' care, which was delivered by local authorities and charged for. This too would be exploited by successive governments after 1980 to erode the comprehensiveness of NHS care. And the power granted to hospital consultants meant that some were better able to argue for their specialties than others, and there was always a perception that some services, in particular mental health and geriatrics, were marginalised.

But of all the weaknesses that Bevan's unavoidable compromises involved for the NHS, the most serious in the long run was undoubtedly the retention of private practice. The existence of a parallel system of private medicine is something British people take for granted (although it astonishes visitors from Canada, for example, where for-profit hospitals and a two-tier, public and private, system are in effect illegal). In 1948 hospital consultants agreed to become salaried employees, but they extracted from Bevan the right to continue with their private practice as well – a policy the Treasury quite liked, because it helped reduce the pressure to keep raising their salaries. So patients with money, or with employers willing to provide them with private medical insurance, have always been able to opt out into private treatment (and then opt back into the NHS again when the costs get too high – or if something goes wrong). The sight of hospital consultants offering patients the expedient of a private clinic appointment in order to be bumped ahead of the NHS queue for investigation and treatment soon became familiar. NHS legislation stipulates that private care should never be at the expense of NHS care, but this has never been strictly enforced.

The system was thus far from perfect, but it delivered what it had promised. Its essential philosophy – that care should be a continuum from prevention to cure, from antenatal services to palliative care and bereavement services, and free to all as a right – remained intact, and became embedded in the ethos of its staff. Its architects and administrators overcame the political buffeting and behind the scenes set about developing a system of planning and organisation that became the model for much of the rest of the world. The overriding principle that secured comprehensiveness, universality and equity was integration, which was designed into both funding and organisation. Because district and regional health authorities were responsible for co-ordinating all administrative and information functions, major gains in efficiency and major improvements in provision could be achieved and wasteful duplication could be avoided. Regional health authorities had responsibilities for planning services for large populations of one million to five million. Their functions included data collection, development of information systems, co-ordination of screening programmes and child health systems, and organisation of services for rare or very expensive treatments such as infertility, blood transfusion, transplantation and genetic screening. District health authorities, on the other hand, were responsible for meeting the health care needs of populations of 250,000, providing district general hospital services and community-based services such as district nurses and other specialist care. This meant that the NHS was exceptionally economical to run. No other Western country could match its costs, largely because no other country had so radically eliminated market mechanisms within the system: with the exception of external suppliers and private patients there was no invoicing and so no payment of bills. The integration within the NHS system depended on the rejection of the idea of health care as a commodity. Above all it depended on designing systems of funding and organisation that promoted redistribution, risk pooling, risk sharing and equity (see Chapter 4).

THE DRIVE TO RECOMMODIFICATION

But by the late 1970s the NHS – the most cost-effective health service in the world – was being labelled 'unaffordable'. The 'new right' was on an offensive to 'roll back the state' and open up public services to private enterprise and the NHS with its million workers was a prime target. And in the mid-1980s a further factor came into play. The US health care industry was in the doldrums. It needed to find new markets and had identified Europe, with its high spend on health care but low penetration by commercial providers, as an unopened oyster. But European health care systems were all well protected against market predators. In the UK the funding and organisation of health services were particularly well integrated through area planning and national ownership and control. Only the pharmaceutical and biotechnology industries had a significant presence. The private sector needed an entry point to tap into public health care revenues. In 1991 this was finally provided by the Conservative government's institution of the so-called internal market.

This was a seminal moment for the global health care industry: the UK's path-breaking socialised health care system turning its back on its founding vision and embarking on an experiment in markets. The NHS, after serving as a model for comprehensive and universal health care, was now to become a laboratory for market mechanisms – mechanisms that would in turn be exported for use across the other welfare states of Europe. By 2003 there was not a single European country that had not embarked on a similar process of market-driven reform. Belief in the superior efficiency of the private sector became the new shibboleth. The costs – in terms of a progressive loss of comprehensiveness, universality and equity, as well as in terms of money – were brushed aside. The Labour Party, which had created the NHS, became dedicated to its destruction.

2

THE REAL COST OF
MARKET PRESCRIPTIONS

Visitors to NHS hospitals today are struck by the way more and more of their forecourts look like cramped shopping malls, cluttered with outlets of W.H. Smith and café chains. NHS hospitals have become yet another outlet for the fast food industry, adding to the very problems of obesity and heart disease that the NHS exists to combat. This transformation began after the introduction of the internal market, when hospitals were expected to supplement their income from commercial retail rentals and private patients. NHS income-generating schemes are also behind the contracting-out of hospital car parking, TV and phone services to companies such as NCP and Patientline. It is now more expensive to park your car at the new out of town PFI Royal Infirmary Edinburgh than at Edinburgh airport. Phone charges are exorbitant: calls to patients are charged at peak rates, and the use of television costs patients on average £16 a week, or one-fifth of the basic pension – a particularly regressive charge, since pensioners and the poor tend to need more hospital care than other people. Ward staff resort to charity and emotional pressure, politely encouraging other patients to top up their phone and television viewing accounts on their discharge from hospital for the benefit of poorer patients. No mechanism is available to patients and their families to challenge these new costs. The only choice is to pay up or go without.

Costs like these are obvious, but they are only the tip of an enormous cost iceberg. With every new market 'solution', new costs are incurred, but most of them are hidden. They are both monetary (i.e. involving additional expenses) and non-monetary (i.e. services contract or disappear). What used to be free and universally available becomes scarce, and then available only for payment. This chapter spells out the crucial connection between market 'solutions' and their real costs, a connection that is key to the significance of the chapters which follow.

THE COSTS OF THE INTERNAL MARKET

Before 1991, hospitals and community services were under the jurisdiction of district health authorities and were accountable to local residents through the health authorities' boards. Every year the health authorities received a block of funding, which was allocated on the basis of a needs-based formula, and from this they had to allocate funds to all the services in their area on the basis of the needs of the residents. Hospitals and community services likewise received their funding in the form of an annual lump sum, agreed in advance with the NHS regional office and the local health authority. There was no invoicing or contracting, although all expenditure was published in detailed annual accounts. GPs had freedom to refer patients to the consultants and hospitals they judged most appropriate. But, crucially, an attempt was made to measure and define the needs for services, and to plan services accordingly. From time to time there was interference by politicians, especially in marginal seats, which distorted allocations and planning decisions, but that was a problem of democratic accountability, not of the planning system itself.

After the introduction of the internal market in 1991 (described more fully in Chapter 3), however, the basis of funding altered dramatically. The link between the allocation of funding and the meeting of residents' needs and service priorities was broken. Instead hospitals were established as financially independent corporations and required to generate enough income to break even. Block funding was abandoned. Now hospitals' main source of income was from contracts placed by NHS purchasers (the health authorities and some GPs, called 'fundholders', who were given the funds to buy elective hospital services for their patients); the rest came from private patients and income generation (described in Chapter 4). The Conservative government under John

Major argued that contracting would allow 'money to follow patients', and so provide more choice. But exactly the opposite occurred.

Hospitals now had to bring in income by negotiation with health authorities and GP fundholders, in competition with other hospitals. This meant that they had to establish elaborate systems for pricing and invoicing in order to negotiate with potentially dozens of different purchasers with different buying powers and purchasing requirements. Some purchasers, for instance, only wanted certain kinds of care, such as heart surgery, while others might want to buy a range of care such as services for older people. Hospitals had to check to see which kinds of care they would be paid for and which they would not. Health authorities and other fundholding purchasers had to decide where they would place contracts and how much they could afford and for what. Patients could now only go where purchasers held contracts for care. Some health authorities placed strict limits on what care would be provided, and so their hospitals had to seek authorisation before proceeding to treat certain categories of patients. These patients were chiefly those with complex and especially expensive-to-treat conditions, for example people needing heart and kidney transplants, or those with chronic severe conditions such as anorexia or bulimia where special placements were needed. These became known as 'extra-contractual referrals', patients whom clinicians could not treat until they had received prior authorisation from the purchaser. Choice was in fact not expanded but curtailed by the internal market.

Increasingly health authorities began to draw up criteria for *denying* care, often with little clinical involvement in the decision-making. For example Lambeth and Lewisham health authority drew up draconian criteria limiting access to varicose vein surgery – despite the fact that severe varicose veins can be very painful, especially for workers such as flight attendants, restaurant staff or supermarket checkout staff. Local residents in one of the poorest areas of England now had no choice but to pay privately for treatment, or go without.

Other health authorities began to restrict access to care for certain treatments and conditions, using the extra-contractual referral mechanism. The famous Child B case illustrated the conflicts and dilemmas that arose because of the separation of power and responsibility for care under a market system. Child B had acute lymphoblastic leukaemia and had had a bone marrow transplant. The doctors felt further treatment would bring no further benefit and indeed would cause great distress to the child and decided not to undertake any more. The parents appealed to Cambridgeshire health authority, which took the view that this was a cost–benefit issue – that the resources could be better used elsewhere – and refused to authorise treatment. The High Court, however, upheld an appeal by the parents on the grounds that the health authority had not explained its decision-making process. But the Court of Appeal over-turned this decision, saying that it was unfair to expect bureaucracies to explain the basis of their decisions. An anonymous benefactor made avail-able the £75,000 needed for private treatment, but the child died eight months later. The point was that clinical decision-making was now open to challenge, using the apparatus of the internal market.[1]

Meanwhile many GP fundholders, who had in general received more generous funding in relation to the number of their patients than had health authorities, were negotiating preferential access for their patients. The result was a postcode lottery in which people had different levels of access to care according to where they lived and who their purchaser was. For the first time, hospitals had to take cognizance of where patients came from and check that the funding from contracts would cover their care. Every month the hospital management team and board would review the performance of contracts to establish which had over- or under-performed on payment. For the first time in the history of the NHS, clinical need was being subordinated to payment performance. Hospitals would plan to treat or refuse patients according to the performance of the relevant contract, i.e. the ability of the purchaser to pay. Often, towards the end of the financial year, wards and theatres would be closed if the hospital had overspent, to enable it to save on staffing costs. If no more contract income was due, patients' admissions would be deferred until the next financial year. Some hospitals found their budgets and services so destabilised by unpredictable fluctuations in funding that health authorities had to bail out some services at the expense of others. Other hospitals simply 'rationalised' services and closed down wards.[2] Health authorities themselves were also unable to manage their finances predictably, and many fell into deficit.

In this way the running of hospitals switched from a focus on planning services to meet patient needs, to a focus on contract performance and income – and the denial of care (see Chapter 4). The introduction of contracting also required a whole new bureaucracy. Each hospital and community service had greatly to expand their departments of finance, in order to set prices and conditions for treatments and to handle multiple contract negotiations and monitor contract performance. Administrative costs almost doubled, but as NHS budgets barely kept pace with inflation much of the increase had to be met from clinical care budgets.

The unequal purchasing powers of health authorities and GP fund-holders meant that patients living in the same street with the same condition could find themselves on different waiting lists and with access to different treatments, depending on what 'their' purchaser was prepared or able to pay. This was most obvious in drug prescribing, where some purchasers rationed drugs more keenly than others – for multiple sclerosis and fertility treatments, for example. People increasingly began to wonder if their GPs were acting in their patients' interests, or in the interest of their budgets. GP fundholders, who were allowed to retain the surpluses from their budgets to invest in their practices (including in the practice premises, which often belonged to them), would also try to persuade some of their patients to use private health insurance or would write private prescriptions in order to save on the practice's NHS budget.[3] Some fundholders, to make a political point, had a deliberate policy of excluding patients they considered high-risk. Many GPs felt deeply uncomfortable with their new role, and and even the normally conservative British Medical Association (BMA) mounted a vigorous campaign in defence of the NHS against the introduction of the internal market.

But while patients and doctors were very unhappy with the changes, the fact that the costs of operating in this new bureaucratic thicket meant cutting other elements out of the NHS was not apparent, at least not to patients. In an already seriously underfunded system, health authorities and trusts needed to divert money from clinical care into the new contracting, monitoring and accounting bureaucracy. NHS hospitals were typically required to find 'efficiency' savings of 3 per cent in their budgets every year, which meant no new posts and the squeezing out of innovation.

'Efficiency' savings also translated into new forms of outsourcing of catering, security and ancillary staff. This provided a less politically

damaging way of cutting staff wages and of reducing terms and conditions than trying to dismantle national terms and conditions of service
that had been agreed with the unions. Outsourcing could be done on the
basis of local decisions, and the government could pass off any resulting
staff disputes as merely local problems. The outcome was the erosion of
the wages of the lowest-paid and most vulnerable hospital staff, and a
corresponding decrease in the quality of the outsourced services.[4]
Moreover these deficiencies are not blamed on the companies supplying
the services. The government argues that poor cleanliness ratings are the
responsibility of the hospitals concerned, because proper monitoring of
the cleaning contracts should prevent it. In practice, 'proper monitoring'
would consume all the resources supposedly saved by outsourcing.

The costs of the structural reorganisations involved in adopting the
internal market, and the inequitable distribution of NHS funds to
purchasers, meant that the whole system was placed under serious
financial strain. More drastic measures were soon required to meet the
rising deficits of NHS bodies. Managers were deflected still further
away from providing care to focus on another kind of 'savings': estate
'rationalisation' programmes. Like an impoverished gentlewoman, the
NHS turned to selling its dowry – its land and assets, or 'estate'. From
1991 onwards, hospital and health authority mergers became commonplace, driven by the need to sell off estate in order to balance the
budgets. For example during my five years of working in a south
London health authority the authority underwent two mergers, with
some staff changing site three times over that period. The mergers
allowed the authority to cut staff and services and dispose of land and
buildings. But even these mergers and sales were not enough. The next
step was to close entire hospitals.

In 1996, for example, the recently merged health authority of
Merton, Sutton and Wandsworth, serving a very mixed inner-city population, wrote a proposal called 'The Rivers Run Dry', in which it
declared that because it had insufficient funding it would have to close
Queen Mary's district general hospital at Roehampton. The health
authority had tried everything to make the savings it needed to balance
the books; now nothing short of closing a major hospital would do. The
task that then faced them was to persuade the clinicians and the public
that this was necessary. The public had already seen several smaller

hospitals in the area close over a ten-year period, but this was the first major acute hospital to be axed. Management consultants were called in to help with the potential adverse publicity. Special strategy groups were established to work on 'scenario planning' and to present the decision to the public as a technically neutral analysis.

The health authority found allies in the Royal Colleges of Physicians and Surgeons. After a visit to the hospital the Royal Colleges withdrew training accreditation for junior doctors in paediatrics – in other words they declared that Queen Mary's Hospital Roehampton no longer offered adequate training for junior doctors in this field. Withdrawal of training accreditation for junior staff means that in effect a hospital can no longer operate an emergency service for the specialty, as it then hasn't enough staff to provide 24-hour cover. The result is a domino effect, first on other specialties and finally on the viability of the whole hospital. At Roehampton the effect of withdrawing accreditation for paediatrics was to close the Special Care Baby Unit, which destabilised the hospital's ability to provide a maternity service and children and baby services. This meant that a full Accident and Emergency service could not be sustained, which in turn meant that training and accreditation for surgery and general medicine would be affected. This process was replicated across the country following other trust mergers.

It was not the responsiblity of the Royal Colleges to think of the system as a whole, or in terms of population needs. Their mandate is only to preserve the standards of medical training. But they are also dedicated to the interests of their specialties and to protecting their relationship with the government; as a result they sometimes fail to take a responsible look at the wider impact of what they do. An important example of this is the contradictory position the Royal Colleges took over what size a district general hospital should be. The Royal College of Surgeons wanted 'centres of excellence' serving catchment populations of 500,000 people so as to provide a wide range and high volume of surgical conditions for the benefit of trainee surgeons, whereas the Royal College of Physicians advocated hospitals serving populations of only 150,000.[5] In each instance it was a question of the numbers of cases needed to sustain a good service seen from the point of view of the training needs of the doctors concerned, to the exclusion of the full range of the health care needs of the population affected.

But the Roehampton decision lay ultimately with the government. It could have intervened to stop the Royal Colleges withdrawing accreditation, or altered the outcome. But it found their intervention most convenient. That alternative solutions were possible with the right sort of political will was never presented as a possibility to staff or the public. For example hospitals can provide 'cross-cover' to each other; with the right sort of planning, services do not have to be closed. But the government could now present decisions to close hospitals and services as being driven by the medical profession, in the interests of patient care and quality. Members of the public felt they had to bow to the inevitable. They were never given the real reasons that led to their local hospitals and services being closed, namely the high cost of introducing market mechanisms in a context of static or even shrinking resources.

There was considerable local opposition to hospital closures. Across the country numerous campaign groups sprang up, some with more success than others, but the government was able to present the closures as little local difficulties and with a few significant exceptions the campaigns eventually fizzled out. The exceptions were in Kidderminster, Glasgow, Kent & Canterbury, and most recently Northern Ireland. In Canterbury, where there was strong public support for the local hospital, the community health council took the government to a judicial review, but lost. These campaigns became national news when local doctors took a prominent part in them, becoming politicised in the process. Particularly effective was the success of the leader of the Kidderminster campaign, Dr Richard Taylor, when he stood as an independent in the 2001 election and unseated the local Labour MP, David Locke, a would-be junior minister. This success was repeated in the Scottish elections in May 2002 when Dr Jean Turner, a retired GP standing as an independent, won a Glasgow seat over the threat to close Stobhill hospital. The government's announcement in February 2003 that it would no longer close smaller local hospitals was a notable acknowledgment of the power of popular mobilisation,[6] although by then much of the damage had been done, and a year later a fresh programme of closures of small hospitals in Oxfordshire was announced. It looked as though in reality small hospitals would still be closed whenever public attention was sufficiently focused elsewhere.

THE COSTS OF THE PFI

When Labour came to power in 1997 no Private Finance Initiative (PFI) hospital-building contracts had been signed, and in public Labour appeared ambivalent about the policy. Harriet Harman, Labour's first minister of social security was on record as describing it as a 'Trojan horse for privatisation'.[7] But one of Labour's first acts was to push through the legislation required, and within months the first wave of PFI hospital deals had been signed. Alan Milburn, as Secretary of State for Health from 1999 to 2003, liked to call it the largest hospital-building programme in the history of the NHS. The reality is that it was also the largest hospital closure programme. The PFI was paid for by major cuts in clinical budgets and the largest service closure programme in the NHS's history.

Under the PFI, which is described in more detail in Chapters 3 and 4, the government goes to a consortium of bankers, builders and service operators which raises the money on the government's behalf, in return for which they get the contract to design and build a hospital and operate the supporting facilities for thirty or more years. But responsibility for paying back the debt and paying interest and the shareholders' profits rests not with the Department of Health but with the hospital, which must pay for them out of its annual budget for patient care. And the PFI rapidly proved to be much more expensive than normal government procurement, for three reasons. First, the private sector cannot borrow as cheaply as the government can. Second, in any PFI scheme the consortium must generate profits and pay dividends to shareholders who have invested in the PFI hospital. Third, costs include the costs of servicing the new bureaucracies, both within and outside the NHS, which are needed to make and monitor all the contracts and subcontracts involved, costs which would not be incurred under normal government procurement.

Until 1991, NHS regional and district planning teams had undertaken the planning of new hospitals: estates, architecture and procurement expertise was concentrated at the levels that provided the greatest efficiency. But the 1990s had seen the closure of these departments; under the internal market, responsibility for planning and for funding new investment passed to individual hospital trusts. Leaving aside the fact that individual hospitals were in no position to undertake an overview of local residents' health care needs, they also lacked the necessary expertise for service planning. Now each hospital had to purchase advice from firms of accountants, lawyers and management consultants (many of the latter having established their own companies after being sacked from the old NHS regional and district departments). This approach meant each hospital having to reinvent the wheel.

The NHS thus incurred huge new costs in the shape of the fees charged by lawyers, accountants and management consultants for drawing up and negotiating complex contracts with a life of thirty years, as well as the costs of raising finance and of planning services. The Department of Health estimated the total of all these costs at between £1 million and £4 million per project; in some cases they amounted to over 8 per cent of the total cost of the hospital.[8] Large amounts of senior hospital management time now also had to be devoted to planning and managing individual schemes, and added to these costs were those incurred by the private sector: the costs of finance and management, which added about 40 per cent to the total cost of each project. These were costs that would not have been incurred under public sector procurement. The new Dartford and Gravesham PFI hospital, for example, cost £94 million to build, but this figure escalated to £115 million when the costs of fees and finance were added in.[9] while the costs of privately financing Worcester hospital increased the bill to the hospital by almost £30 million.[10]

All these costs had to be added to the total debt, to be repaid over thirty years by the hospital trusts concerned. This created an 'afford-ability gap' between the private PFI consortiums' monthly charges, and what the hospital trusts could afford to pay – as if one's rent doubled or tripled overnight while one's income stayed the same. Thus in Dartford and Gravesham the cost of servicing capital rose from 6 per cent of the annual budget to 32 per cent.[11] These escalating costs alarmed the Treasury and the Department of Health, but the government had staked too much on the project to back off, the scheme having been previously bailed out with hidden subsidies – receipts from land and asset sales, internal capital transfers, and Treasury-funded 'smoothing mechanisms'. But this was still not enough, and the hospitals concerned were left with no alternative but to close the gap by paring away services. In the first wave of PFI hospitals this amounted to an average reduction of 30 per cent in beds, and in some schemes a 25 per cent cut in the salaries budget, mainly for nursing staff.[12]

To achieve these cuts the main planners of new PFI hospitals, the outside management consultants – no longer working within the framework of the NHS, and so less likely to be inspired by its founding principles – became mercenaries, their technical skills now serving the market.[13] Objective planning methodologies were jettisoned in favour of a more or less exclusive focus on the affordability of each PFI scheme. Services and beds were cut to fit the costs, and justified by acrobatic leaps of faith in increased levels of 'throughput', to be achieved by new 'performance targets'. In Edinburgh one chief executive talked of 'turning away trade' – i.e. turning away patients – in order to arrive at the needed 25 per cent reduction in bed numbers. Many of the schemes assumed that the average length of a stay in an acute hospital could fall from around four days to just over one, despite the fact that the average length of stay was beginning to rise again; this was because the scope for pushing patients into day case surgery was reaching its limits, and the remaining inpatient beds were now occupied by sicker patients requiring more intensive and longer periods of care.

The connection between the PFI and all these problems is concealed from the public by the complexity of the transactions involved, and the rhetoric of the government and the pro-PFI lobby, but it is entirely real. The cuts in hospital operating budgets that have had to be made to fund the higher costs of PFI hospital building are the real reason why across the NHS hospitals' cleaning and catering standards are reduced, NHS-provided transport is no longer available, waiting times obstinately refuse to fall, seriously ill patients are parked for hours on trolleys waiting for a bed, and cuts are made in the ratio of nurses to patients and consequently in the quality of clinical care.

THE COSTS OF PRIVATISING LONG-TERM CARE

The internal market raised costs in other sectors as well, and notably in long-term care. The 1990 NHS and Community Care Act made local authorities responsible for long-term care, leaving the NHS with only a residual role in the care of older people. To gain access to NHS long-term care services, individuals now had to demonstrate entitlement by meeting a set of eligibility criteria and jumping over a number of hurdles (described in Chapter 6). But this required the creation of another new bureaucracy. By 1994 each of the 100 health authorities employed staff, usually nurses (a scarce resource in the NHS), to draw up and apply 'continuing care criteria' which would restrict entry to NHS long-term care and shunt costs to patients and carers. The placement of each patient now had to be authorised and funding for it agreed between the local health authority and social services. Where there was uncertainty each case would be reviewed by a panel of doctors, nurses and social workers; in other words, health care professionals were now having to spend time discussing the denial of care, rather than giving it.

The criteria for receiving long-term NHS care were very tough, and depended on the care places available in each area. The results were great variation in access to care and the deliberate erosion of the core NHS principle that health care should be universally available to all. The policy of shunting responsibility to local authorities allowed the NHS to continue closing services and selling off associated land and buildings. Health authorities faced with mounting deficits set about selling what was left of what had once been extensive long-stay facilities, including the much-loved small cottage hospitals. The Oxted and Limpsfield War Memorial Hospital in east Surrey, for example, served extremely frail elderly and chronically sick people, many of whom were completely bed-bound and entirely dependent. The hospital was a tranquil oasis in a green setting, with lots of land that developers had their eye on. Although it was badly in need of refurbishment, the atmosphere and care were of the highest quality. The authority desperately looked for ways of transferring these services to the private sector, using management consultants to advise on 'scenario planning'. Local people fought a fierce campaign to try to keep the hospital open, but to no avail, and the same story was played out across the country. The land associated with long-stay hospitals, among them many huge institutions for the care of people with mental illnesses, was sold off for golf courses, luxury homes and supermarkets, while most of the care and services that were provided in them simply disappeared.

Politicians presented these service closures as moving care into 'the community'. But the main result was that older people got a much-diminished level of access to the NHS. As a result of the NHS divesting itself of this responsibility for older people, the expertise and knowledge that had been built up through the specialty of geriatrics were sidelined, becoming very marginal elements within the rapidly shrinking acute hospital sector. Many older people now have to go without the essential care they need. Their care is now the responsibility of local authorities, which do not have the knowledge and expertise required. A study of older people in Barking, for example, showed that before their transfer to nursing and residential care homes more than 90 per cent of residents had been diagnosed as having serious clinical depression. Subsequent case note reviews showed, however, that despite their high levels of need fewer than 10 per cent received the treatment and support they required.[14] Only GP services were provided.

The UK was once famed for its pioneering work in the care of older people – the specialty of geriatrics had a worldwide following. But local authority social service departments, which now became responsible for this work, had little knowledge of the benefits of geriatrics, and were inclined to see any attempt to introduce it into the care of older people as 'medicalising' the process of ageing. But this is a misunderstanding, which ignores the extent to which geriatrics is as much about prevention as cure. Geriatricians do not see decline as an inevitable consequence of old age: a geriatrician would not see incipient blindness or deafness, for example, as an inevitable result of ageing, and would expect many stroke victims to make significant recovery given expert rehabilitation involving speech therapists, etc.

There were still further costs as the buck passed down the line in the new long-term care regime. Care formerly provided free by the NHS was now the responsibility of cash-strapped local authorities, which sought to shift the costs, if they could, to patients and carers. Local authorities were encouraged to introduce their own systems of eligibility criteria, euphemistically called 'care planning'. They too now had to create new bureaucracies whose remit was to define and apply exclusion criteria for services, on the basis of ability to pay. 'Care planning' became a strategy of limiting the provision of services, 'targeting' those most in need of care. Prevention, and preventative care and support, which had been a fundamental philosophy of NHS social care departments, was now out of the question; the focus was on late intervention, not assessment, to minimise the risk of legal challenges to the local authority. For all the rhetoric of 'care in the community' the numbers receiving community-based care from local authorities dropped dramatically – for instance between 1995 and 2000 there was a 22 per cent drop in the number of people receiving home help, and between 1995 and 1998 there was a 32 per cent drop in the number of people receiving meals on wheels.[15] Local authority services now targeted only the most frail and needy, most of whom would have received a far wider range of expert services under the jurisdiction of the NHS, and local authorities provided little or nothing for large numbers of others.

'Care in the community' also meant a greater shift of long-term care provision to the private sector under contracts that were not subject to public scrutiny of the financial disadvantages involved, as Chapter 6 shows. But there were other big unforeseen, or at least undeclared, costs of bringing in the private sector. For example at the height of a financial crisis in the Merton, Sutton and Wandsworth health authority it was discovered that in its eagerness to dispose of estate and beds at Springfield Hospital, a large psychiatric hospital, it had placed five-year contracts with Cumberland Nursing Home in Mitcham owned by a large for-profit chain, Care UK, which provides places for the elderly mentally ill. However bed occupancy at Cumberland Nursing Home was at one point less than 40 per cent. At the time I estimated that this represented a loss of some £400,000 a year being paid for unfilled beds, money that was going straight to the private sector with no return whatsoever. But government guidelines required the health authority not to relax the eligibility criteria and admit more patients for fear of the longer-term revenue implications after the contract had expired. No one knows how much money has been wasted in this fashion by both health and local authorities all over the country.

Means-testing for services has meant that many people choose to make their own arrangements for personal care, rather than having to pay, in any case, for whatever placement the local authority finds for them. But then they are left with no come-back if their chosen private care providers fail to provide. The concept of long-term care as a right or entitlement has truly disappeared.

Worse still, the Labour government not only endorsed the Conservatives' removal of long-term care from the NHS, but has also used the resulting blurred boundary between health care and 'personal care' to start curtailing people's right to other kinds of health care by reclassifying it as 'intermediate' care. This concept was initially invented to describe care for people in hospital who no longer needed the facilities of an acute hospital, but who were not ready to return home. This 'intermediate' care would be paid for by the NHS, but in facilities that would be provided primarily by the 'independent' (for-profit or voluntary) sector, chiefly in nursing homes which would be upgraded for the purpose (see Chapter 3).

But 'intermediate care' proved to be a new mechanism for restricting access to NHS care: in January 2000, for the first time in the history of the NHS, time limits were introduced for NHS care, and later embodied in legislation.[16] 'Intermediate care' is now free for the first six weeks. After that it becomes a joint NHS and local authority responsibility, and may be charged for. With this change, health care free at the point of service ceased to be an inviolable principle.

The impulse behind this policy was bound to surface in other ways, and sure enough in December 2003 the government announced that it planned to extend it to some of the most vulnerable groups in the UK: foreign patients and failed asylum seekers. As a result of the new rules, 'foreign' patients and those suspected of being failed asylum seekers would now have to demonstrate their eligibility before they could receive health care.[17] It proposed that entitlement would no longer be a right of all UK residents. According to a press report, in future 'suspect' patients would have to prove their entitlement to care by providing proof of residency in the form of bank records or council tax pay-books.[18] According to the government the aim was to put an end to what it called 'health tourism', which it claimed was costing the NHS some £200 million a year. But there was no evidence to support this claim. The early results of a study in Newham – an inner-city area with a high density of immigrants and refugees and asylum seekers – showed that over a three-month period only 17 patients were not eligible for NHS treatment, and the total cost to Newham was £32,000 – i.e. a bare fraction of its £300 million annual NHS expenditure.[19] As the well-known health economist Alan Maynard commented – before embarking on instituting a complex and socially divisive new administrative policy the government really needed to check whether the evidence supported it.

THE EMERGING HEALTH SERVICE – NO LONGER COMPREHENSIVE, UNIVERSAL OR FREE

The architects of the NHS were well aware of its inherited weaknesses, and the resulting problems they were designing into it, but they always hoped that political leadership, responding to popular opinion, would allow these problems to be designed out at a later stage. And so in spite of everything the NHS was a remarkable success. Health care became what its architects had envisaged: a right of citizenship, covering all health needs and increasingly equally available in all parts of the country; and with the exception of prescription charges, introduced during a financial crisis in 1951, free. On top of this the NHS was amazing value for money, precisely because it was thoroughly integrated and rationally planned, with a workforce highly committed to its public service ethos.

But chronic underfunding and persistent attacks from the Right meant that after 1979 integration and needs-based planning were displaced by market ideology. The internal market weakened the immunity of the NHS to market forces; in particular it weakened integration by uncoupling the resources given to health authorities from the services provided, creating entry points for private operators of all kinds to tap into NHS funds. Within the NHS itself, introducing the logic of the market turned existing weaknesses and tensions into open fractures, susceptible to colonisation by new market pathogens. When Labour came to power in 1997 the process of disintegration and market transformation was already well under way.

Under New Labour, instead of reintegration and the restoration of the NHS's founding values, a series of new market solutions were prescribed. As a result, costs were driven up, not down; bureaucracy continued to expand, instead of decreasing; inequities of all kinds were aggravated, not reduced, and new inequities were created; more services that had been free were to be charged for, or would largely disappear from the NHS, to be provided only by the private sector, for those able to afford them. Comprehensiveness and universality became things of the past. Inequalities of all kinds flourished. The resulting decline would foster yet more discontent, and eventually market forces would overwhelm the NHS's defences. Health care moved increasingly rapidly away from being a right, back towards being a commodity – as it had been before 1948.

3

PRIVATISING THE NHS: AN OVERVIEW

background

problems

Although elements of the privatisation process pre-date the Thatcher government, 1980 was when privatisation began to be official policy. By then the NHS had suffered thirty years of serious underfunding and a good deal of administrative reshuffling. Its hospitals were often dilapidated and some still dated from the Victorian era. Staff shortages were common and there were long waiting times for non-urgent hospital treatment. Pay for nurses and support staff had been kept low and morale was wearing thin. But a more equitable geographical distribution of resources had gradually been achieved, and the NHS's founding principles of comprehensive, universal care, equally available to all on the basis of need, not ability to pay, continued to prevail. What is more, the country's overall health statistics compared well with those of other industrialised countries, not to mention those of the USA, which spent twice as much per head on health care (see Tables 3.1–3.3). And in spite of its weaknesses the NHS remained extremely popular.

But in 1980 the Thatcher government began radically reshaping the NHS, fragmenting its structures, significantly reducing its coverage, and undermining evenness of provision from one district to another, while financial targets increasingly displaced health care needs as the focus of concern. Twenty-three years later the NHS had abandoned to the private sector almost all long-stay inpatient care, all routine optical care and most dental care, and multinational corporations from across the world were being invited to take over the running of 'failing' NHS

Table 3.1 Health expenditure per capita (£) and as per cent of GDP (in brackets)

	1960	1970	1980	1990	2000
OECD average	26 (4.5)	74 (6.0)	346 (7.3)	839 (8.7)	1,500 (10.0)
EU 15 average	15 (4.0)	53 (5.4)	333 (7.3)	837 (7.8)	1,193 (8.7)
USA	51 (5.1)	145 (6.9)	506 (8.7)	1,553 (11.9)	3,057 (13.0)
UK	19 (3.9)	41 (4.5)	234 (5.6)	555 (5.7)	1,126 (7.1)

Source: OHE, *Compendium of Health Statistics 2002*

Table 3.2 Life expectancy at birth (years)

	1950–55	1960–65	1970–75	1980–85	1990–95
OECD	63.2	66.4	67.8	70.0	72.2
EU 15	64.8	67.6	68.7	70.8	72.9
USA	66.2	66.7	67.5	70.9	72.2
UK	66.7	67.9	69.0	71.0	73.7

Source: OHE, *Compendium of Health Statistics 2002*

Table 3.3 Infant mortality rates per 1000 live births

	1960	1970	1980	1990	1998
OECD	37.6	28.3	17.5	10.7	7.0
EU 15	43.2	31.1	19.4	11.1	7.4
USA	26.0	20.0	12.6	9.2	7.2
UK	22.5	18.5	12.1	7.9	5.7

Source: OHE, *Compendium of Health Statistics 2002*

hospitals and to provide routine NHS surgery in private Treatment Centres. The government had also just finished pushing through legislation under which most if not all NHS services, including hospitals, will eventually become more or less independent corporations, run on business lines. This chapter tells, in outline, the story of how this came about.

1980–1990: FINANCIAL STRANGULATION AND THE END OF COMPREHENSIVENESS

Mrs Thatcher's initial aims were relatively limited: to curb spending on the NHS, weaken its public sector unions, and reduce the power of hospital consultants, who were seen as obstacles to efficiency and economy. It was an article of faith (which New Labour would later adopt with the fervour of converts) that only managers with private sector entrepreneurial values could make the NHS efficient – a faith backed by a doctrinal 'revolution' concerning public administration. The 'new public management' became the dominant ideology in public administration textbooks, emulating a distinctly idealised model of private management, including the doctrine that public bodies, like private companies, should concentrate on their 'core' activities and 'outsource' the rest.[1] This provided a good rationalisation for curbing the power of the large public sector unions in the NHS. So from the early 1980s onwards NHS hospitals, like local authorities, were required to put more and more non-clinical tasks, such as cleaning, laundry and catering, out to contract with the supposedly more efficient private sector, and frail elderly people in need of long-term care were transferred out of NHS hospitals into private nursing or residential homes.

The Conservatives were convinced that all public bodies were wasteful, lacking the whip of competition, and this particularly included the NHS, which accounted for some 14 per cent of all government spending. The Treasury agreed. It had always sought ways to curb the NHS budget, seeing it as inherently tending to grow out of control.[2] The consensus of expert opinion was that the NHS needed annual real funding increases of about 2 per cent to keep level with growing needs, but through the mid-1980s it received about 1 per cent.[3] Instead NHS *'efficieny saving'*

hospitals were told to find 'efficiency savings' of 3 per cent a year. Given that health care is by its nature labour-intensive, the scope for achieving savings through greater efficiency was actually limited; in practice 'efficiency savings' meant cuts in staff and services in some areas to make possible urgently needed growth in others.

From the early 1980s onwards the Conservatives initiated two other structural changes, in addition to outsourcing of non-clinical hospital work: the introduction of general management of hospitals and cutting back the coverage provided by the NHS.

The first change followed a report in 1983 by Sir Roy Griffiths, a supermarket manager invited by Thatcher to review the running of hospitals. He thought the hospital sector, managed by administrators and senior consultants on the basis of 'consensus', was in a state of 'institutionalised stagnation'. He could not understand how it could run without someone like himself in charge. This was summed up in a carefully crafted soundbite: 'In short, if Florence Nightingale were carrying her lamp through the corridors of the NHS today she would almost certainly be searching for the people in charge.'[4] What the hospital service needed was general managers with overall control.

The Griffiths report was accepted and over the next few years 'chief executives' supplanted senior hospital doctors in the management of hospitals. The number of general or senior managers in the NHS rose from 1,000 in 1986 to 26,000 in 1995, and the proportion of total NHS spending consumed by administration more than doubled, from 5 to 12 per cent.[5] The new managers became even more powerful with the introduction of the 'internal market' in the 1990s. The new hospital trusts (see page 41) now had to undertake a wide range of administrative, financial, legal and technical tasks that had formerly been performed by NHS regional offices or district health authorities; the trusts had also to recruit and service new boards of governors, as well as to meet the vast increase in 'transaction costs' involved in contracting. In due course some managers came to be appointed on short-term contracts, sometimes with 'performance-related' pay. Managing a hospital soon ceased to be seen as the pinnacle of a career. Now it was just one stopping point among others on the way to the top in a wider management job market. A new 'business culture' was installed in hospital policy-making.

non-clinical employment in NHS

Installing general managers also helped to drive the second major policy change of the 1980s – 'contracting out' or 'outsourcing'. The 'core' activities of the hospital service were defined as 'clinical' and were to remain 'in-house'; all other activities, from meal services and cleaning to laundry and maintenance, now had to be contracted out to private service providers. As a result, non-clinical employment in the NHS fell dramatically throughout the eighties, from 260,000 in 1981 to 157,000 in 1990 (and went on falling, to a low of 120,000 in 1994).[6] But the results were not impressive. At the levels of funding the NHS had become used to, the outsourced services could only be made to yield profits by cutting the number and pay of staff, and so reducing quality. A 2001 study of outsourced hospital work in east London found that almost all those interviewed earned less than £5 an hour. Staff taken on directly by the outside companies typically earned about 20 per cent less than equivalent NHS staff and had much-reduced other benefits, from holidays to pensions;[7] indeed this was the chief factor permitting outside firms to make a profit. While costs may have been cut (the evidence is disputed), any gains were at the expense of employment and service standards.[8]

Throughout the NHS the turnover of support staff rose and hospital cleaning standards fell while the poor quality of hospital meals became notorious.[9] Incredible as it might seem, 10 per cent of seriously ill patients were found to have suffered malnutrition while they were in hospital.[10] In November 2000 a 'Better Patient Food Initiative' was launched, with a budget of £40 million, under the supervision of the American TV food programme presenter Lloyd Grossman; but without tackling the inherent problems of factory cooking and minimal food budgets no significant improvement was possible.

Managing the outsourcing contracts, and monitoring their performance, often consumed more administrative time than had previously been needed to manage the services in-house. Perhaps the main effect of outsourcing, however, was further to replace the professional culture that had previously prevailed in NHS hospitals with a business culture focused less and less on medical values and more and more on the bottom line of hospital and health authority accounts.

The third main change in health policy in the 1980s was the near elimination of several kinds of care from NHS coverage: routine optical services, a great deal of dentistry, and most long-term inpatient care for the frail elderly and people suffering from chronic diseases. In other words, the NHS's founding principle of 'comprehensiveness' of care was drastically eroded. The government also declined to fully fund the increasingly important provision of terminal care in hospices, which remain dependent for half their cost on charity.

Routine eye examinations ceased to be offered free under the NHS in 1989; opticians now charged fees. This was justified on the grounds that people could afford the fees, but it led to a two-thirds drop in the rate of examinations.[11] NHS dentistry was cut back, partly by big increases in the fees already charged to patients, but also by stealth. Dentists, like GPs, were mostly 'independent contractors' with the NHS. So from the later 1980s onwards the government simply capped spending on dental services until fewer and fewer dentists were willing to provide their services at the NHS rates, and more and more started declining to take new patients 'on the NHS'. By 1999 more than half of all dentistry was paid for by patients. Fewer than one-third of all dentists worked exclusively on NHS terms, mostly in low-income inner-city areas. By 2002, 51 per cent of spending on dental care was accounted for by private provision.[12] The NHS had thus already become a 'residual' dental service, offering a basic treatment mainly for children up to age sixteen and adults who are unable to pay the full cost of private treatment – a model, in fact, for the rest of the NHS as the private health care industry envisaged it.[13]

The elimination of long-term care from the NHS, with the closure of most NHS long-term care beds, was well under way in the 1980s, and is described in Chapter 6. In the barest outline, the Thatcher government decided to take long-term care out of the NHS and create a predominantly private long-term care industry. Local authorities were made responsible for ensuring that residential care was provided for all those in their area who needed it. Unlike NHS care, local authority care was charged for, subject to a means test. Central government funding from the Social Security budget was made available to cover the fees for those who could not afford to pay – but only if they were placed in privately owned care homes, as opposed to those operated by local authorities themselves. A private care home industry was thus brought rapidly into being, and by 2003 provided 69 per cent of all long-term care places.[14]

Patients who had been in long-term care in NHS hospitals and were transferred to private homes in the 1980s and 1990s had their fees paid for out of special transitional funds, but people newly requiring long-term care became responsible for paying for it themselves, if they had sufficient resources. A distinction was made between 'nursing' care, which was narrowly defined but still covered by the NHS, and 'personal care' – washing, feeding, etc. – which had to be paid for. (As one GP put it, 'nursing' now covered roughly anything above the waist. Everything below it was 'personal care'.) Despite public anger at these developments, only the new Scottish Parliament voted to provide all personal care free under the NHS in Scotland. In England and Wales, people who depended entirely on state benefits and local authority funding found themselves placed in care homes where the fees were lowest, often receiving seriously inadequate care.[15] In effect, for the most vulnerable people in society the NHS principle of equal care regardless of ability to pay had been abandoned.

But in spite of all these reductions in the coverage of the NHS, and the abandonment of its founding principles that this involved, the NHS still could not cope with the level of financial constriction it was being subjected to. Capital spending continued to be minimal. As Chapter 4 shows, a new hospital renewal plan launched in 1962 was never fully implemented. Only one-third of the projected 224 schemes were completed; one-third were partially completed, and one-third were never started. Capital spending was invariably the first victim of the incessant sterling and balance-of-payments crises of the 1960s and 1970s, and during the Thatcher and Major years public spending was even lower on the government's agenda. Between 1980 and 1997, only seven NHS capital schemes of any kind costing more than £25 million were completed.[16] The ratio of doctors and hospital beds to population lagged more and more behind those of comparable countries (see Table 3.4). Waiting times increased, both to see a GP, and even more, to see a specialist; and after that, to receive hospital treatment if it was needed. Both GPs and hospital staff experienced rising levels of stress as they struggled to maintain services in face of growing demand without the necessary resources.

Table 3.4 Doctors and hospital beds per 100,000 population, 1999

	Doctors	Hospital beds
France	328	834
Germany	355	920
Italy	589	487
UK	176	413
EU 15 average	375	630

Source: *Eurostat Yearbook 2003*, pp. 101–2

1990–1997: THE 'INTERNAL MARKET'

In 1987 the Conservatives' continuing financial squeeze finally brought the hospital sector close to collapse, and in face of an unprecedented public protest by the presidents of the Royal Colleges of Physicians, Surgeons and Obstetricians, as well as the NHS nursing and support staff unions, Thatcher was forced to change course. At this point she adopted, with remarkably little forethought (and no consultation inside the NHS), the idea of an 'internal market' promoted by Alain Enthoven, a US Defense Department economist who had latterly been employed by the leading US arms manufacturer, Litton Industries. The NHS was now split into 'purchasers' – the health authorities and some GPs – and 'providers' – that is, the hospitals and community health services, and GPs. The aim was to make NHS managers and doctors behave more like businessmen and women. Hospitals and community health services were organised into more than 400 autonomous 'trusts', legally obliged to break even by 'selling' their services to the 'purchasers' at the prices specified in the contracts drawn up with them. This reorganisation, implemented in the early 1990s, was accompanied by two significant short-term funding increases – one of 6 per cent in real terms in 1992-93, and another of 4 per cent in 1994–95 – but most of this extra money was absorbed by the costs involved in establishing the new system of separate 'purchasers' and 'providers', and the costs of all the contract negotiations, billing, contract monitoring and enforcement, etc., of the internal market itself.[17] The Treasury continued to believe that the NHS could be made more efficient by being kept under financial pressure. Hospitals were still expected to make 'productivity savings' – that is, to cut costs – by 3 per cent a year.

The internal market never achieved the efficiencies it was supposed to achieve, above all because it was politically impossible to allow hospitals actually to compete with each other and let the less competitive ones go out of business, as would happen in a real market.[18] Whole districts could not be left without hospitals. But the planning capacity of the NHS was nevertheless run down. Health authorities were reduced in number and scale, shedding and devolving to trusts their responsibilities for human resources, planning and payroll, and dispersing the expertise of their staff; while some of the new hospital trusts, being too small to handle these functions efficiently on their own, were obliged to resort to expensive outside help from management consultants.

The sums did not add up and services did not improve. By 1996–97 one-third of all hospital trusts were failing to meet at least one of their financial targets, and waiting times for non-urgent treatment (especially 'elective' surgery to deal with painful but non-life-threatening conditions) failed to fall, and even rose slightly.[19] But the fragmentation of the hospital service into hundreds of separate trusts with purely financial obligations, and the 'purchaser–provider' split, set the NHS on a radically new path. These measures began the destruction of the NHS's capacity to plan and distribute resources on the basis of the health needs of the population, and opened the way for the later moves towards the privatisation of clinical services.

The new trusts were conceived on the model of commercial companies, run by chief executives with boards of directors consisting chiefly of businessmen.[20] Senior hospital consultants became Clinical Directors of the various specialties, with cash-limited budgets related to the number of 'finished consultant episodes' (or 'FCEs') achieved; in other words, hospital doctors became subject to increasingly tight central management control and had less and less influence on policy. They were also no longer free to speak out on policy issues: they were now employees of the trusts they worked for, not the NHS, and often had 'gagging' clauses in their contracts that prevented them from making any public statements critical of the trust. (One trust chairman, Roy Lilley, even declared that doctors' duty to their trust came 'before the professional duty to the patient'.)[21] Trust boards were appointed by the Secretary of State for Health on the advice of the local health authority and were effectively unaccountable; they were obliged only to publish an annual report and hold one open meeting a year (which chief executives tended to regard as a waste of time).

Although the NHS Executive could issue 'guidance', which trusts were in practice bound to follow, and had general oversight of trusts' performance, the dynamic of change in the NHS now began to shift decisively from needs-based planning on behalf of the residents of a given area to a purely pragmatic process of change, whereby trusts tried to adapt their performance to their financial circumstances. Local conditions varied, often leading to a wide gap between a trust's income and the demand for its services, and there was no automatic mechanism for balancing the two. Local health authorities did what they could to offset the effects of these inherent mismatches, but with limited success.

These difficulties were aggravated by 'capital charging', which was also introduced in 1991. The idea behind this move, which was to be applied to all public services, was that if trusts had to pay interest and dividends on their capital assets (land, buildings and equipment) they would use them more efficiently. The trouble was that trusts had inherited widely differing amounts and quality of capital assets. A trust might operate two hospitals on valuable inner-city sites, with high market values, and hence find itself paying a high capital charge to the Treasury without being able to recoup the cost by charging the local health authority or other purchasers correspondingly more for its services. It might be able to win some temporary respite by selling off genuinely surplus assets, but it could not reduce costs by moving to a cheaper site unless new capital was made available for a new building. Trusts caught in this situation were forced to try to reduce costs by neglecting maintenance and cutting services (which made waiting times worse and increased the stress on their staff). A more popular solution among the new chief executives and chairmen of trusts was to sell the existing site and build a new hospital on a 'greenfield' site outside the city centre, using private finance (see below). In practice this invariably increased costs, instead of reducing them. Either way, the result was that serious discrepancies developed between localities in the level of services provided to patients.

GP 'fundholding' added a further complication. In the name of making hospitals more responsive to patient needs, and giving patients more 'choice', beginning in 1991 large general practices were invited to 'hold' and manage the budgets for all 'routine' hospital treatment for the patients on their lists. The scheme was gradually extended to smaller and smaller practices until by April 1997, 55 per cent of GPs in England had become fundholders, and up to 14 per cent of all hospital and community health trust income was being derived from contracts with GP fundholders.[22] GPs who became fundholders in the later 'waves' increasingly did so to avoid their patients being discriminated against by those who had already become fundholders, as hospitals responded to the more demanding conditions that the first fundholding GPs were often able to set for the patients on their lists (shorter waiting times, especially). In other words, a two-tier hospital service was emerging – or three-tier, if we include the private patients treated in NHS hospitals.

Indeed, treating private patients also became much more significant in the 1990s, thanks to the 'internal market'. Using taxpayers' money to provide special beds for private patients makes little sense, yet in London and some other centres, where there were significant numbers of people with private medical insurance, it looked like a cost-effective way for some hospital trusts to earn additional income to help close their deficits, and many created separate private patient units, staffed by NHS nurses, for the purpose. In 2003 there were some 3,000 private beds in NHS hospitals, 1,300 of them in seventy-six special Private Patient Units, chiefly in London, separate from and offering superior accommodation to ordinary NHS wards.[23]

The internal 'quasi-market' also led to the quasi-pricing of more and more activities. One of the great original strengths of the NHS was that all its activities – from public health to family medicine to heart transplants – were integrated, the cost of one activity becoming a saving in the cost of another. For example, preventative care, or early hospital admission, can save having to provide more complex and expensive care later. Savings of this type – so-called 'externalities' – can only be taken into account when costs are integrated. They disappear, in the sense that they are no longer taken into account, when costs are counted only for individual units or departments. The remarkable cost-effectiveness of the NHS, 'a system in which wealth was distributed according to need, and nobody knew the cost of anything', hinged significantly on service integration and cost-sharing.[24] Moreover no part of the NHS had to charge, or pay charges to, any other part, which also kept its transaction costs to a minimum.

The internal market progressively destroyed these advantages. Now every clinical directorate in a hospital, such as cardiac or orthopaedic surgery, was supposed to 'cost' every significant activity it undertook, and the Department of Health took to using the national average of such costs as 'reference costs' against which to measure the degree of efficiency each hospital was achieving. The rewards of integration were lost as each organisation within the NHS was increasingly obliged to assess all its costs as if it stood alone, like a small or medium-sized business, covering its own financial, administrative, personnel, capital and other costs. And in spite of all the talk within hospital trusts of the importance of 'care pathways' – for instance how heart surgery must be integrated with cardiac rehabilitation services and ongoing aftercare – the drive to cost individual 'treatments' separately militates strongly against this.

Of course there are better and worse-run parts of any service, however it is organised. But instead of enquiring case by case why some hospitals seemed to have much higher costs, and confronting the complexity of the inherited structures and widely differing local conditions that are usually responsible, health economists and health ministers found it easier to believe that higher costs were mainly due to bad management, and that 'badly performing' hospitals could be made more efficient by threats, and if necessary by coercion – by sending in 'hit teams' of outside managers to take them over.

A further impetus to fragmentation and the loss of a rational basis for planning and allocating resources was that outsourcing was extended from support services like cleaning and catering to more sophisticated services such as information technology, accounting and service planning. By the early 1990s hospital trusts and, increasingly, health authorities too, could no longer turn to the NHS Executive's Regional Offices for help, these having been run down (they were finally abolished in 2001). Now they had to rely on outside management consultants, whose quality varied and whose expertise, such as it was, seldom compensated for their lack of close knowledge of the institutions or communities being planned for. Health authorities too were shedding more and more of their experienced professional staff, while covering larger and larger areas as they merged with each other in search of 'economies of scale' (their numbers fell from 192 in 1982 to 100 in 1997).

In theory the outsourcing of planning was supposed to be a more efficient use of NHS resources. In practice the record suggests that the loss of planning capacity inside the NHS has cost it dearly, even in simple cash terms. The advice of outside consultants led the first wave of Private Finance Initiative (PFI) projects to adopt unsustainable targets for reductions in bed capacity, that then had to be expensively revised. All the projects involved outside consultants, at a cost of between £1 million and £4 million per project,[25] and all of the projects proved more expensive – in some cases spectacularly so – than the consultants originally estimated.[26]

The hidden costs of outsourcing may be almost as great. A glance at the considerations that go into drawing up a contract with a private sector provider makes it very clear why large firms exist in the first place – they want to avoid the massive transaction costs involved in outsourcing everything.[27] The sheer complexity of establishing in fine print all the elements involved and all the contingencies that may arise, and the resources needed to monitor performance, need to be offset by very large gains if outsourcing is to be worthwhile. And what advocates of public sector outsourcing often overlook is the fact that when large firms outsource, they usually take care to do so with external providers who are in a relatively weak position *vis-à-vis* themselves, and with competing alternative suppliers always available. In the case of outsourcing by the public sector service providers, this is rarely possible. In the case of a hospital there is often no alternative local supplier to turn to, at least in the short run, and continuity of service is essential. As a result the penalties specified in the contract for poor performance are rarely enforced because the costs to the hospital of changing suppliers would be so great. The real risks arising from poor perform-ance by a cleaning or catering firm, for example, not to mention poor performance by an outside pathology laboratory, are actually borne by patients, not the contractors.

Outsourcing information technology has had a further serious effect: more and more of the information is now collected at public expense by outside firms under contract. The resulting databases can increasingly be accessed only on payment of fees – fees that are prohibitively large for independent researchers – or by NHS bodies that agree to pay an annual subscription of several thousand pounds to the firm in question. For example CHKS (Caspe Healthcare Knowledge Systems) Ltd. collects and analyses hospital trust databases and makes the comparative analyses they undertake available to the trusts involved for an annual subscription of £5,000. But only half of all trusts are clients, and not all the clients' data are included in the results, which are in any case 'anonymised'. This means that reliable and comprehensive data and analyses on which to base future public spending on health services are less and less available to NHS planners, not to mention independent health policy analysts. The effects of policy changes on the population are thus becoming harder to discover, while policy is driven more and more by the short-term financial and commercial imperatives that the local units of a 'decentralised' NHS are operating under.

The privatisation of information is particularly damaging when supply constraints also tend to overwhelm rational planning. Through-out the 1990s the funds made available for delivering NHS services continued to be squeezed, as we have seen. The long-term decrease in the average length of stay in hospital, made possible by new therapies, including 'day surgery', had levelled off (see Table 3.5), but hospitals were kept under intense pressure to cut costs and increase the 'throughput' of patients, so that throughout the 1990s the number of available beds continued to fall (Table 3.6). Such overall figures do not reveal the impact of cuts on particular services and areas. For this, detailed local information is required, which is less and less available. If the necessary data are collected at all they remain at the level of hospital or primary care trusts and are not brought together centrally.

And while effective public accountability based on publicly accessible NHS-wide data was being eroded, patients were increasingly encouraged to look at the NHS not as a valuable shared legacy from the Keynesian welfare state, but as a collection of businesses offering things to consume. A significant indicator of this was the 'Patients' Charter' introduced by the Major government in 1991, spelling out a range of standards that the NHS was supposed to reach, such as to see patients within fifteen minutes of their arrival at an Accident and Emergency

Table 3.5 Average length of stay in NHS hospitals, England

Acute Inpatient Finished Consultant Episodes

Year	1991	1992	1993	1994	1995	1996	1997	1998	1999	2000	2001	2002
Days in hospital	6.1	5.7	5.5	5.4	5.2	5.1	5.0	n/a	n/a	n/a	n/a	n/a

Ordinary admissions, all causes

Year	1991	1992	1993	1994	1995	1996	1997	1998	1999	2000	2001	2002
Days in hospital	16	14	12	10	9	8	8	8	8	8	8	8

Source: OHE, *Compendium of Health Statistics 2003–2004 & 2002*

Table 3.6 Average daily available NHS hospital beds, total (UK) and acute (GB)

	1951	1960	1970	1980	1990/91	2000/01
Total hospital beds, UK ('000s)	543	560	536	458	338	242
Per 1,000 population	10.8	10.7	9.6	8.1	5.9	4.1
Acute hospital beds, GB ('000s)	n/a	182	171	158	142	129
Per 1,000 population	n/a	3.6	3.2	2.9	2.5	2.3

Source: OHE, *Compendium of Health Statistics 2003–2004*

department. The Charter did not confer enforceable rights – it gave patients 'the option of complaining (if these standards were not met) but little else'[28] – but it did help to foster higher expectations, and it fed into the wider consumerist currents which have encouraged a sharp increase in litigation against the NHS.

The amounts of compensation awarded by the courts have also increased dramatically. The net present value of the expected awards in outstanding claims in England alone rose from £1.3 billion in 1996–97 to £2.6 billion in 2001 – close to 5 per cent of the entire NHS budget for England; the expected cost of incidents that had already occurred but for which claims had not yet been made raised this total to £3.9 billion.[29] Of course people should be compensated for injuries resulting from clinical negligence. But the cost to the NHS is substantial and one is bound to wonder whether it is not partly the other side of the coin of 'efficiency savings': failures of care caused by faster 'throughput', over-stretched staff, smaller ratios of highly trained to less-trained staff, etc. (The Infection Control Nurses Association and the Health Protection Agency, for example, said that hospital cleanliness 'had not been helped by over-reliance on poorly paid contract cleaners with no allegiance to the NHS'.)[30] And it is a cost the NHS budget will have to continue to cover, even though the increasing fragmentation of the NHS, and the inclusion of for-profit surgical service providers of unknown quality, has the potential to drive it up further still.

1997–2000: CONTINUED FRAGMENTATION UNDER NEW LABOUR

When Labour returned to office in 1997 its policy towards the NHS was influenced by powerful national and international forces that had begun to gather strength in the 1980s and became more and more influential as the 1990s wore on. One was the famous 'tax aversion' of the elec-torate, brought about by the bitter campaign waged by the Conservative Party and the right-wing press against the 'overblown' welfare state: Labour came to power committed not to raise income tax and not to exceed the Conservatives' published spending plans for the next two years. In this situation, remedying the NHS's chronic underfunding was out of the question. There was even less chance of tackling the NHS's building maintenance backlog, which by then amounted to over £2 billion, or of modernising the total NHS 'estate' (the Wanless Report would later put the total cost of doing that at an additional £40 billion over twenty years).[31] The financial starvation of the NHS continued.

But the pro-business stance of Blair and Brown – plus the decision to transfer authority to set interest rates to the Bank of England – was politically successful in the short run. The City's hostility was signifi-cantly reduced. Important personal and financial ties were established with businessmen such as David Sainsbury, Geoffrey Robinson, Bernie

Ecclestone and Michael Levy, and an accommodation was reached with Rupert Murdoch's right-wing *Sun* newspaper. But this meant that policy now had to be conducted in line with business interests. No significant Conservative privatisation was reversed and the PFI – which had its first and most extensive trials in the NHS – was pursued enthusiastically, even when it proved far more expensive than traditional procurement. Outsourcing of ancillary hospital services was maintained, and Labour not only left long-term care largely in private hands but actually increased the pressure on local authorities to privatise both the care homes they still owned and the domiciliary services they provided in the community.

Tony Blair's first Minister of Health, Frank Dobson, was a well-liked and competent minister. Unfortunately for him, his two years in office, 1997–99, were the years during which the Chancellor of the Exchequer, Gordon Brown, had pledged to keep public spending within the Conservatives' previously published plans. Dobson did promptly announce the end of the NHS 'internal market', suggesting that this would save £1 billion a year for spending on 'front-line' services, but he was not allowed to abolish the division of the NHS into purchasers and providers and its associated bureaucracy. All he could do was to restrain the pro-market zeal of some hospital chief executives by issuing a letter authorising them to send patients for treatment in private hospitals only where the NHS hospital's capacity was being used to the maximum, and to report all such instances to the Department of Health.[32] And since he could make no significant improvement in NHS funding he could make no real impact on waiting times or the quality of service provision. In 1999 he agreed to resign his cabinet post and stand as Labour's candidate for Mayor of London, and after losing badly to Ken Livingstone disappeared for a while from the political stage. But before he left office Dobson presided, however reluctantly, over two initiatives inherited from the outgoing Conservatives that would prove hugely significant: the establishment of Primary Care Groups, and the signing of the first wave of contracts for building new hospitals under the PFI. Both measures radically accelerated the fragmentation of the NHS and its permeation by private capital.

Primary Care Groups/Trusts

When Dobson announced the end of the internal market – retaining the 'purchaser-provider split' but replacing 'purchasing' with 'commissioning', in which only broad categories of services were specified in the 'contracts', and for three years at a time instead of annually – he also announced the end of GP fundholding. But in reality he made all GPs into fundholders through his reorganisation of the UK's 30,000 GPs into some 480 'Primary Care Groups', or PCGs, which would later become Primary Care Trusts or PCTs. Each PCG/PCT was to comprise all the general practices and community health staff in a given locality, with average populations of 100,000. As with hospital trusts, the number of PCTs would also decline through mergers. By 2003 there were just 303, covering average populations of 170,000. At first, as PCGs, they only 'advised' the local health authority on the commissioning of hospital services for the patients in the practices they comprised. But in 2002 their graduation to trusts status was abruptly accelerated – i.e. they all at once became PCTs – and in 2003 they became responsible, in theory at least, for spending 75 per cent or more of the total NHS budget for their areas, i.e. including the budget for 'secondary' (general hospital) care.

While the idea of a 'primary-care-led' service had been part of the rhetoric of successive governments since the inception of the NHS, making GPs and community health doctors and nurses responsible for most of the budgets of district general hospitals was something else. Most GPs lacked the knowledge and skills to take on this responsibility, having received no training in the complex policy and economic issues at stake. If hospital trusts lacked the epidemiological and other planning expertise previously available from health authorities, most PCTs lacked it even more. In effect, transferring control of the NHS budget to GPs and other community-based health staff meant that the principle that the best possible health care should be offered everywhere alike was seriously jeopardised.

The Department of Health continued to issue 'guidance' to PCTs, and also to allocate their budgets; and the twenty-eight Strategic Health Authorities, which replaced the district health authorities in 2002, could give them instructions so as to try to ensure that they met their performance targets.[33] It seemed, in fact, that large hospital trusts, with their concentrations of management skills and senior clinicians, and their local monopolies of provision, were unlikely to be inclined to accept orders from PCTs, whatever the PCTs' nominal control of hospital budgets might appear to imply. The new regime was more likely to be a system of local single-seller markets, with funding actually allocated according to decisions made by, and in the institutional interests of, hospitals. Indeed many PCTs lacked the professional resources even to fulfil some of their own most basic independent tasks, such as public health, as Chapter 5 shows.

PCTs also became responsible for the prescription budgets of all the general practices in their area. Hitherto health authorities had urged GPs to limit their prescriptions to an approved list of drugs considered effective and affordable, but had refrained from telling them what they could and could not prescribe, and had eventually picked up the total bill. Now, however, each PCT has a fixed drugs budget and has to ensure that its local GPs stay within it. This is a significant downloading of risk onto relatively small 'risk pools' – the pool of people who share the risk of becoming ill. If a PCT happens to have an unusually high proportion of patients who need very expensive drugs, some of these patients may have to do without, or other services will have to be reduced.

The Private Finance Initiative and Public–Private Partnerships

When Frank Dobson left office in 1999 PCGs were still being organised, and the first group of PCTs came into being only in April 2001. But the Private Finance Initiative was a different story. The PFI had been conceived in the early 1990s, partly in response to the recession in the building industry, which had very close ties to the Conservative Party then in office. Under the PFI, 'special purpose vehicles' or SPVs – i.e. consortia of construction companies, facilities management companies and banks – would raise money, by issuing shares and borrowing, to build, own and operate public service premises such as hospitals. Hospital trusts would lease the buildings, complete with maintenance and other support staff, under contracts lasting twenty-five to thirty years or even more. As well as offering rich returns to the private sector the PFI was presented as a way of getting new buildings without raising taxes, at least in the short run (and also not having to show the cost as part of the public debt – an advantage that the Accounting Standards Board later curtailed). The public would still be paying for the hospitals, but payment would be deferred, like hire purchase (but minus the purchase, since when a PFI hospital contract comes to an end the land and buildings will in most cases still belong to the private owners, not the NHS). Moreover the annual payments by the hospitals were to come out of their existing operational budgets, forcing them to find ways to become more efficient too.

But it took considerable time to work out the details in such a way as to make the private sector willing to participate, and in 1996 the necessary legislation still had not been put before parliament. The fate of the PFI therefore hung in the balance as the Major government, mired in scandal, headed for defeat by Labour in the 1997 election, and Labour's attitude to it became one of the tests of its pro-business credentials. Within weeks of taking office Labour announced its support for the PFI, and NHS hospital building projects were its first and most-publicised examples. In spite of damaging expert criticism of the PFI in terms of its cost, efficiency and effects on services, and in spite of widespread public hostility as its failures in one field after another became apparent, Labour continued to pursue it with extraordinary determination. The government's 2002 White Paper *Delivering the NHS Plan* said that in addition to the thirty-four PFI hospital projects already completed or signed for, a further fifty-five major hospital schemes would be carried out 'mostly through the PFI'.[34]

Yet the government's commitment to the PFI (now renamed Public–Private Partnerships, or PPPs) became more and more paradoxical. By the year 2000 the intellectual case for the PFI had been widely discredited, to the point where the government declined to debate it and resorted to merely denigrating its critics. It gradually became clear that the real motives behind it lay elsewhere: partly in the Labour leadership's anxiety to keep business support, and their new-found preference for businessmen and women over public sector managers, and partly in their calculation that an opening up of all countries' public services to private sector provision through the General Agreement on Trade in Services or GATS (see pp. 60–61 below) was inevitable, and that by advancing faster and farther in this direction than most other countries they would give British firms a competitive advantage. The European Commission's enthusiasm for PPPs, especially for the EU's new member states, offered a particularly promising potential market.[35] In other words it was a foreign policy as much as a domestic one.

The case against the PFI is that (a) it is more expensive than public financing; (b) it locks the public sector – in this case, hospital trusts – into paying for buildings over periods of 30–60 years, during which time needs may change radically; (c) it changes the focus of planning from the health needs of local populations to the needs of hospitals and private capital; and (d) in the case of the NHS (though not in all other parts of the public services, such as schools) the cost of paying for the new privately built and operated buildings has to be met out of operating revenues. Therefore the new buildings have to be smaller so that bed numbers and staff can be reduced. These reductions are driven by financial necessity, not by any analysis of health care needs. It is clear that Treasury officials thought that forcing NHS hospital trusts and health authorities to pay for new hospitals out of current revenues was a good way to make them more efficient. The result was that 'performance targets' were built into PFI plans – targets for the number of 'finished' consultant episodes (a proxy for admissions), rates of throughput of patients, bed occupancy rates, etc. – that had no conceivable basis in past or foreseeable trends.[36]

A significant role in this was played by the much more commercial culture that the internal market had established within the NHS. Plans now tended to be based on corporate 'mission statements' and 'visions', rather than assessments of need and projections of resources. Population-based planning, involving epidemiology and other public health specialties, was disparaged; as we have already seen, the planning capabilities of health authorities and of the NHS Regional Offices – their teams of economists, architects, engineers, surveyors, public health doctors, etc. – were dispersed. The professional medical ethos that used to underpin hospital management gave way more and more to 'entrepreneurialism', and in some cases to a distinctly 'macho' management style.

The upshot was that as PFI hospitals began to come on stream, bed shortages became even more acute, waiting times failed to get shorter, and staff turnover increased as more and more was demanded of fewer and fewer people. The once-outstanding effectiveness of the NHS had been sacrificed to parsimony and market dogma for so long that Britain now began to lag behind some other comparable countries in survival rates for serious conditions such as heart disease and cancer, and even in rates of infant mortality.[37]

Already in 1999 mounting evidence of a nationwide shortage of hospital beds had prompted the Secretary of State, Frank Dobson, to institute a national beds inquiry for England inside the Department of Health. Reporting in 2000, the inquiry concluded that in the immediate future 3,000 more hospital beds were required nationally.[38] Yet it is a measure of the overall loss of planning rationality that in arriving at this conclusion the inquiry did not take into account the further loss of beds that would continue to occur as more and more 'downsized' PFI hospitals came on stream. It almost looked as if Dobson's successor Alan Milburn saw the national beds inquiry mainly as a sop to public concern, while the Treasury's drive to cut bed numbers continued unchecked.

The mechanisms of the PFI have been so much discussed that only a brief account should be necessary here. Requiring all NHS hospitals to pay the Treasury 6 per cent annual interest on the value of their capital assets from 1992 onwards – a 'capital charge' – was presented as a way of making the NHS use its capital assets wisely. In practice, however, as we have already noted, it meant that hospital trusts that had inherited expensive assets they could not easily sell off were suddenly loaded with costs that they could not pass on in full to the 'purchasers' of their services (the health authorities and GP fundholders and, later, the PCTs).

Nonetheless, the principle having been established that NHS trusts had to pay for their capital assets out of operating revenue, it was not such a big step to go on to say that instead of paying interest on their capital assets to the Treasury, hospital trusts could pay an annual fee to a consortium of private companies for making hospital buildings available to them for a period of 30 to 60 years. But the cost of a new building built via the PFI was significantly higher than if it had been built with public finance, since a private consortium's cost of borrowing was on average between 1 and 4 percentage points above the cost of public borrowing. Together with the other costs associated with private finance this meant that the 'availability' fee paid to the private consortium (i.e. the annual payment for the use of the buildings) was much higher than the 6 per cent annual capital charge previously paid to the Treasury – in fact for the first wave of PFI hospitals it was between two and three times higher.[39] To meet it, either more money had to be found out of the local NHS operating budget, or costs had to be reduced. As this 'affordability' problem grew, the chief solution was to cut costs by making the new hospitals smaller.

The average reduction in bed numbers in the first wave of PFI hospitals was 30 per cent, while budgets and numbers of clinical staff were cut by up to 25 per cent.[40] In the PFI 'business plans' these cuts were justified in terms of 'new models of care', whereby significant amounts of health care would be shifted from acute hospitals into 'community-based' services – including 'intermediate care' provision for inpatients no longer in need of acute hospital care, but not yet ready to go home. But whereas health authorities often specified that the trusts' PFI plans should assume that such services would be provided, they did not spell out what these alternative services would be, let alone how they would be paid for, and in most cases they did not materialise.

The government justified the increased capital costs involved in PFI projects – and the service reductions they entailed – by saying that they would 'drive' new efficiencies, making them ultimately cheaper than publicly financed projects, and that their greater cost also represented risks transferred to the private sector consortia – risks formerly assumed by the NHS, which now had to be paid for. These arguments have been shown to be largely groundless. The alleged inefficiency of public sector provision, resulting in cost overruns, was based on wild exaggeration; for example, rather than taking the actual average cost overrun of 6–8 per cent in NHS projects during the 1990s, PFI business plans assumed that cost overruns in public sector procurement would be anything from 12 per cent to as much as 34 per cent (in the Norfolk and Norwich PFI plan). And the discount rate adopted by the Treasury – which gives the total payments that hospital trusts undertake to make over 30–60 years in PFI projects a lower 'net present value' than the expenditures that would be made over the few years of the construction period in traditionally procured projects – was eventually acknowledged to have been deliberately set at a figure that gave the PFI an apparent cost advantage.[41]

As for risk transfer, in one case after another it has been shown that risks are not really transferred. The consortia that raise the money get 'triple A' ratings from the credit rating agencies, and pass the risks that are supposed to be transferred from the public sector on to the building companies and facilities management companies to which they contract out the work. Whether or not risks are really transferred can only be judged when things go wrong. In practice the costs almost always fall on the public because the service cannot be allowed to collapse.[42] Often no provision has been made in the contract to ensure that the private consortium is really liable for the risks in question (for example the consortium building a PFI hospital in Carlisle was supposed to be bearing £5 million worth of risk that the targets for clinical cost savings would not be met, but the contract made no provision for them to have to pay anything if that happened).

By their nature, the PFI's effects are long-term because the contracts are long-term. New hospitals have been built, more expensively than if they had been publicly financed in the traditional way, and for this reason they have usually been kept small, so as to minimise these costs, regardless of local health care needs. North Durham PFI hospital, for example, costing £97 million, was built with too few beds to handle local demand. As a result the hospital trust was forced to divert money intended for service improvement to pay surgeons to treat NHS patients in nearby private hospitals 'to stop waiting lists spiralling out of control'. In nearby Bishop Auckland, by contrast, a £67 million new PFI hospital was built to replace one already widely recognised to have too small a catchment area for its facilities, yet the hospital trust was now committed to pay for it for a further 27 years. The logical response seemed to be to merge the two hospitals and use Bishop Auckland for the surgery that could not be done at North Durham, but the surgeons involved saw major safety risks in doing this, which would cost yet more money to overcome.[43]

Such problems reflect the fragmentation of the NHS hospital service into competing business units or trusts, each charged with meeting its financial targets within the limits of its inherited capital stock rather than serving the local population's health care needs on a rationally planned basis. Not only are PFI hospitals locking up NHS operating income at the expense of service provision for decades into the future, they are leading to more and more uneven levels of service provision, as trusts with expensive PFI hospitals struggle to balance their books by cutting services to divert funds to meet their PFI payments.

PPPs in primary care

The government's commitment to the PFI or PPPs meant that by 2002 at least 400 major PFI/PPP projects had been completed or were in progress, covering almost every field of public service, from hospitals to schools and government offices and even military facilities. Eventually GP premises became part of the story too, and although this happened mainly after 1999 it is convenient to mention it here. This process was promoted by the Treasury through the Local Improvement Finance Trust, or LIFT, and resulted in GPs increasingly leasing their premises from corporations.[44] Sometimes GPs became shareholders in these companies, while others were owned by private medical insurance companies like Norwich Union and private health care providers like Sinclair Montrose and Westminster Health Care. So both primary care and hospital care are now increasingly provided in corporate-owned premises; through its involvement in the provision of GP practice premises the private health sector is becoming more closely linked to many of the new PCTs, which as we have seen are in theory responsible for spending 75 per cent or more of the NHS's budget.

Moreover, PPP contracts have been moving from a focus on providing public service infrastructure to providing public services themselves, often under the title 'strategic service delivery partnerships'. In other words, it is no longer just ancillary functions like cleaning and building maintenance that are being outsourced but services previously considered part of the NHS's 'core'. For instance the private sector has been lobbying the government hard to privatise NHS hospital pharmacies, and also radiology and pathology services. PCTs will have strong incentives to back this if their commercial partners can persuade them it will make these services cheaper, since they will be paying for them out of the NHS funds under their control – even if all experience shows that savings are invariably achieved (and profits made) by cutting staff numbers and qualifications, and reducing the quality of services provided.

Cost-shifting to patients

Another rather likely effect of the web of private sector interests that the PFI, PPPs and LIFT taken together are spinning round the NHS is cost-shifting to patients. This arises because personal care services hitherto provided by local authorities, such as care provided to people in their own homes (e.g. meals on wheels or home help), are not free, as NHS services are, but must be paid for by patients, or by local authorities, subject to means-testing. Faced with budget constraints PCTs have an incentive to define services as 'personal services' which patients, or local authorities, must pay for, rather than as 'nursing' services whose costs must be met out of their NHS budget. This could be particularly significant for patients transferred to so-called 'intermediate care' beds in private hospitals or nursing homes under the Concordat with the private health care sector (described below). As we saw in Chapter 2, after six weeks of free 'intermediate' care provided by the NHS, patients who remain in need of such care may become liable to be charged for it.

The situation becomes even more complicated with the new Social Care Trusts that combine both health and social service functions and so involve different sources of funding (some from the NHS, some from the local authority, and some from central government). In this setting patients seem likely to meet increasingly unpredictable demands for fees for services, or parts of services. The eligibility rules can vary from one local authority to another, and the complexity of different funding sources with different rules will make it hard to know one's rights.

The IPPR Commission on the PFI

An interesting postscript to the PFI/PPP story was provided by the publication in 2001 of the report of a 'commission' on the PFI established by the Institute of Public Policy Research, a think-tank closely associated with New Labour. The costs of the commission were met by a group of leading companies with major interests in the PFI – the investment bankers Nomura, the management facilities company Serco, the private medical insurer Norwich Union, the private hospital operator General Health Care Group, and the private health care consultancy KPMG. Moreover the commission's members were drawn predominantly from the banking–CBI–Treasury nexus that had been built up around the PFI.[45] So it was not surprising that although its report made various criticisms of the way PFI/PPP had operated so far, it ended by recommending that PPPs should be extended to the provision of core public services in health, education and local government. It rationalised this by treating all the problems it had identified as transient, points on a 'learning curve', resulting from mistakes in the early stages of the PFI, and by studiously avoiding the evidence that pointed to the problems inherent in the whole concept.

The government, having consistently refused to confront research-based criticism of the PFI (in the manner described in Chapter 7), gratefully endorsed the report's conclusions. It was evidently determined to push ahead with the policy despite growing public dislike of it, and despite the fact that no disinterested observer any longer believed in its official rationale. The reasons for this seemed to be New Labour's continuing need to maintain the support of the City of London. The importance of 'business confidence' was starkly revealed in the aftermath of the Railtrack fiasco of 2001. When the then Transport Secretary Stephen Byers finally decided to call a halt to the company's constant demands for additional subsidies, and put it into administration, pressure from the City forced the government to compensate the shareholders, even though the company was effectively bankrupt. It was made clear that future PPP projects would otherwise cost a great deal more, to offset what investors would then see as greatly increased risks. What investors wanted was to be able to make a profit from running public services, financed by tax revenues, at minimal risk.

The impact of trade liberalisation

The government was also influenced by the expected outcome of the current round of negotiations within the World Trade Organisation (WTO) on the General Agreement on Trade in Services (GATS). The negotiations on this trade treaty were secret but leaked memoranda made it clear that tough bargaining, led by the USA and the EU, was likely to lead to a significant opening up of public services to private provision by companies based anywhere in the world. By 1995 over 50 per cent of all foreign direct investment in the major industrial countries was in services. This investment, however, was still predominantly in commercial services, from construction to banking. But during the 1990s pressure built up to open up public services such as health care to international trade on the same lines. Health care was a particularly sensitive field for the Americans, because in Europe it was predominantly publicly provided, while in the USA it was overwhelmingly private. Foreign firms could therefore provide health services in the USA, and between 1990 and 1997 foreign direct investment in US health service provision rose tenfold, whereas the reverse did not occur.[46] Although this amounted to just 1 per cent of the total stock of assets invested in US healthcare, it marginally increased competition.

US health insurance companies and health maintenance organisations (HMOs) like Kaiser Permanente and United HealthCare, facing intensified competition and declining profits in the saturated US market, were anxious to tap into markets abroad, especially the potentially rich markets that would exist if tax-funded health care were provided by for-profit companies. They had persuaded several Latin American governments to let them manage their social insurance health funds, tapping into large streams of tax revenues, virtually risk-free;[47] now they joined in a wider campaign for the privatisation of all public services worldwide via the World Bank, the OECD and the WTO.

The GATS appeared to leave governments free to exempt public services if they wished, and in 1995, when the agreement was signed, only 27 per cent of GATS members opened their health services to market competition. Article 1.3 of the agreement, however, said that the right to exempt public services did not apply if a service was provided on a 'commercial basis', or if it was supplied 'in competition with one or more service suppliers'.[48] Given the opening up to market actors that had already occurred in the NHS (the privatisation of optical and dental services, private provision of long-term care and the accelerating development of PFI/PPP – not to mention the commissioning of NHS treatment from private hospitals), it was clearly going to be hard to argue that the NHS was not provided on a 'commercial basis' or in competition with other providers.

None of this was clear to the public, because the GATS negotiations were conducted in secret. New Labour, however, was reported as giving 'enthusiastic backing' to the list of services being put forward by the EU countries collectively for opening up under the new round of negotiations. The list included water, energy, sewerage, telecommunications and postal and financial services, almost all of which have been privatised in Britain.[49] The government's idea was evidently that this would eventually apply to health services too. While it claimed that health services were excluded from the GATS agenda, its privatising reforms were increasingly bringing them within the ambit of international trade law.

2000–2003: NEW LABOUR'S DRIVE TOWARDS A 'MIXED ECONOMY OF HEALTH CARE'

By the autumn of 1999 Gordon Brown's two-year lock on new public spending had produced a situation in the NHS that resembled the Thatcher-induced crisis of 1987. Public discontent was acute and the government was in danger of forfeiting one of its greatest electoral assets: Labour's identification with the NHS. On the other hand Brown's spending restrictions, coupled with the US-led boom of the late 1990s, had by now produced major fiscal surpluses. So early in January 2000, smarting from universal criticism over the latest 'winter beds crisis', the government pledged to raise spending on the NHS by 6.1 per cent a year in real terms over the next four years – a roughly 30 per cent increase in all, raising NHS spending to 8.2 per cent of GDP (which, combined with private spending on health care, would be close to the current EU average). In return for the increases in pay and staffing and equipment that the new spending would permit, the government wanted pledges from everyone in the NHS to push through 'reforms' in every sector of the service, including the breaking down of professional barriers and the introduction of 'flexible' labour markets. In March 2000 133 senior NHS staff and informed outsiders were hurriedly organised into a set of 'modernisation action teams' which duly endorsed a plan of action that appeared in July. This was the *NHS Plan*.[50]

The NHS Plan

The *NHS Plan*'s goals, though expressed in sometimes overheated prose, were extremely positive, extensive and detailed. By 2010 there would be over 100 new hospitals (including those already under construction), 7,000 more hospital and intermediate-care beds, 500 new 'one-stop' primary care centres comprising dentists, opticians, pharmacies and social workers as well as GPs, and new information technology linking primary care and hospitals. There would be 7,500 more consultants, 2,000 more GPs, 20,000 more nurses and over 6,500 more therapists. By 2005 waiting times for hospital treatment would be reduced from an average of seven months to a *maximum* of six months, and eventually to a maximum of three months. A new system of resource allocation would end the unevenness in primary care provision that meant there were still 50 per cent more GPs per capita in Richmond than in Barnsley, and NHS dentistry would become available 'to all who want it by September 2001'. (This last commitment seemed unrealistic, and so it proved. In August 2003, after a well-publicised incident in Wales when 600 people queued for 300 new 'places' in an NHS dental practice, the government announced that in future dentists would follow GPs and have contracts with their local PCTs, not the Secretary of State for Health.)

According to the *NHS Plan*, National Service Frameworks – general treatment protocols and targets – would be established for more and more illnesses to ensure nationwide achievement of good practice. A Modernisation Agency would spread best practice throughout the system. Hospitals and PCTs would be subject to inspection every four years by the Commission for Health Improvement and rated 'green', 'yellow' or 'red' according to how well they were performing. A 'green' rating would lead to the granting of more autonomy and financial rewards for the hospital management. A 'red' rating would led to more intervention from the centre, including if necessary the installation of new management. (This much-derided colour coding was later replaced by an equally fallible system of 'star' ratings.)

Further privatisation

The *NHS Plan*'s targets were ambitious and made great headlines. What was not so quickly absorbed by the general public was how far the *NHS Plan* would be accompanied by a much more radical marketisation of the NHS, both by opening it up to private providers of health care and by making even the publicly owned institutions of the NHS more and more like commercial companies. It is hard to tell whether the Department of Health's policy team had this radical marketisation of the NHS in mind in July 2000 when the *NHS Plan* was published. They were, as always, under heavy pressure from market enthusiasts in the Treasury, and it seems likely that they already envisaged some mixture of the continental European and the US models, both of which had been advocated in various forms by right-wing think-tanks and many of the department's external advisers. Pressure from both local and global market forces presumably also played a role in what eventually happened. The one body of opinion that was *not* consulted was the British public's. The far-reaching policy changes in the *Plan*, pointing the NHS ever farther down the road to privatisation, had not been put out for public discussion in a Green Paper. And the *Plan* itself, while eventually described officially as a White Paper, was from the first treated as official policy, endorsed by the NHS luminaries in the government-appointed 'modernisation action teams', not as a set of proposals for debate.

An important factor was the situation of the UK private health provider industry which, as we saw in Chapter 1, had not benefited from any of the internal market reforms. The rising cost of health care meant that private medical insurance was now beyond the means of most people; rising insurance premiums also meant that the numbers of people with company-paid medical insurance had stopped growing, and had continued to stagnate even when the economy expanded in the late 1990s (see Table 3.7). From the point of view of the private health care industry, the only solution was to get NHS tax revenues diverted to it, and it lobbied hard accordingly.

Most EU countries, with their mixture of state, independent non-profit and private provision, looked capable of being penetrated in time. The NHS, however, with its universal publicly funded and publicly

Table 3.7 Number of people covered by private medical insurance (millions), UK

1955	1960	1965	1970	1975	1980	1985	1990	1995	2000
0.58	1.0	1.45	2.0	2.3	3.6	5.1	6.7	6.7	6.9

Source: OHE, *Compendium of Health Statistics 2002*, Table 2.22

provided service, free at the point of delivery, still offered fewest openings to the private sector. It became fashionable among market-oriented health journalists and Conservative MPs to refer to its 'Soviet-style' centralised organisation, and to call for it to be broken up into something offering more 'choice', and for people to be able to 'put more of their own money' into the system and let private enterprise 'close the gap between demand and supply'. Behind these calls lay the commercial interests of not only insurance companies and private hospital and nursing home owners, but also nursing agencies, pharmaceutical companies, property development companies, facilities management companies and many more, which were all lobbying hard to erode the boundaries between the NHS and the private sector and get access to the NHS's tax revenues.

One of the boundaries targeted concerned hospital pharmacies. 'PFI is delivering improvements of up to 15 per cent in value for money', declared Tim Stone, whom we met in Chapter 1 advising the government on the PFI, and who was now the 'PFI chair' at KPMG; 'if you got even 10% off the drugs budget at acute hospitals you would be talking about humungous amounts of money'.[51] How humungous savings could be made by privatising hospital pharmacies the press report did not say. The prospect of humungous profits was easier to see.

Such lobbying was helped hugely by the 1997–99 financial squeeze. People increasingly resented waiting longer and longer to see a GP for a consultation lasting on average seven minutes; then waiting months for an outpatient appointment to see a consultant physician or surgeon; and then waiting further months for treatment, especially for 'elective' surgery to deal with painful, if not life-threatening, conditions (e.g. hip replacements), but also, too often, for cancer and other urgently needed surgery. There was also the annual 'winter beds crisis' when, typically, older patients with influenza or chronic conditions aggravated by the cold were forced to wait on hospital trolleys for hours or even days because hospitals no longer had the necessary spare bed capacity.

According to the private health care lobby and the right-wing press, the problem was not shortage of money but wasteful bureaucracy and centralisation. 'Throwing money' at the NHS would not solve it. What was needed was to let private enterprise run publicly financed health care and give 'consumers' the same degree of 'choice' they enjoyed in other spheres of life (in reality, the schemes proposed for increasing choice always turned out to mean better health care for the relatively affluent and a more residual level of care for the rest).[52] New Labour said it remained committed to the NHS and its founding principles, but it accepted the idea that private enterprise was more efficient than public enterprise and responded to all these pressures with ever greater concessions.

The Concordat with the private sector

The *NHS Plan* explicitly renounced what it called the 'standoff' that had existed between the NHS and private health care providers up till then. 'This has to end,' it said. 'Ideological boundaries or institutional barriers should not stand in the way of better health care for patients. ... The private and voluntary sectors have a role to play in ensuring that NHS patients get the full benefit from this extra investment.'[53] The NHS would therefore make a new 'Concordat' with the private sector about providing both critical and elective surgery, and intermediate care for NHS patients, paid for by the NHS. In addition the government would 'explore with the private sector the potential for investment in services such as pathology and imaging and dialysis'. The *NHS Plan* also envisaged involving the pharmaceutical industry in 'the development and implementation of national service frameworks' or protocols for drug therapies for particular conditions, i.e. direct involvement in 'disease management' – a long-held goal of the pharmaceutical industry – rather than relying for their sales on doctors' prescriptions.

In fact the negotiations were already far advanced which led to the signing in October 2000 of a 'Concordat' between the government and the Independent Healthcare Association (IHA). In it the government made 'a commitment towards planning the use of private and voluntary care providers, not only at times of pressure but also on a more proactive longer term basis' which could be 'reflected in Long Term Service Agreements'.[54]

The immediate background to the Concordat was a revealing incident involving Tony Blair. In February 2000, the senior public relations officer at the IHA, Tim Evans, had managed to get into a TV audience for a question-and-answer session with the prime minister. He asked Blair if he had any 'ideological objection to cooperation between the NHS and the private health care sector'. When Blair said no, he told him about Dobson's 1997 letter to NHS trusts (mentioned on page 50) telling them, in effect, only to use private hospitals in exceptional circumstances. Shortly afterwards Blair and his wife were having dinner at London's River Café where they met a journalist whom Blair recognised. Blair asked him if what Evans had told him was true. On being told it was, and after making further enquiries, Blair ordered that Dobson's instruction should be cancelled.[55] Alan Milburn, who had replaced Dobson as Secretary of State in October 1999, then embarked on the negotiations which led to the Concordat.

But there were material reasons behind the Concordat as well. One was that the recently completed national beds inquiry had shown that two-thirds of hospital beds were occupied by people aged 65 and over, and that for about 20 per cent of these – i.e. about 13 per cent of the total number of beds – hospital was not the 'appropriate' place; these elderly patients no longer needed the resources of an acute hospital, but were not ready to be discharged to their homes. What they required was 'intermediate care', 'closer to home'.[56] But because no appropriate facilities existed they had to stay in hospital, 'blocking' beds that were needed by other patients. Since the private nursing home sector had been experiencing declining profit margins from the mid-1990s onwards, it was understandably enthusiastic about the prospect of this potential new source of business.

A second reason was to reduce the waiting times for elective surgery. As we have seen, the growth in the private health care industry had levelled off in the early 1990s, which had left it with large amounts of excess capacity. While NHS hospitals had an average bed occupancy rate of 83 per cent, the average private hospital occupancy rate was less than 50 per cent. The line of least resistance for the government was to invite some of these hospitals to operate on NHS patients who were waiting for surgery – if, the Concordat said, this offered 'demonstrable value for money and high standards for patients'.

But just as few private nursing homes had the facilities to provide NHS standards of care, however 'intermediate', without substantial investment, much the same was true of most private hospitals, which provided a limited but profitable range of elective treatments, using NHS surgeons (and always with the option of moving patients to the nearest NHS hospital if complications arose). So the point was not just to agree to cooperate in general, but to 'signal a commitment' (in the words of the Concordat) on the part of the government to underwrite the necessary investment to upgrade private facilities by entering into long-term contracts with the private sector to pay for clinical services – in effect, shifting more work by NHS consultants from NHS to private facilities, since virtually all private clinical work is done by NHS consultants, outside NHS hours.

By the end of 2003, however, it was becoming clear that the Concordat was largely a dead letter. The prices demanded by the UK private sector had proved so much higher than the cost of equivalent services provided by the NHS that the government could not defend accepting them. Eventually the government declared that it would continue to pursue the privatisation of clinical services, but by opening up the competition to international providers.[57]

Private Diagnostic and Treatment Centres

How far the intermediate care promised in the *NHS Plan* for 'all parts of the country' by 2004 will be provided by the private sector remains unclear at the time of writing. In the acute sector, however, the government has said it expects that private hospitals will perform 150,000 more operations a year for the NHS, a roughly 15 per cent increase in their activity and income. At the same time a high-profile initiative was taken to invite private providers to establish some twenty-seven Diagnostic and Treatment Centres (DTCs, later called Independent Treatment Centres or ITCs) to perform routine hip, knee and cataract operations at an annual cost of £2 billion.[58] The first eleven were to open in December 2003. Together with twenty-five similar centres run by the NHS, it was envisaged that they would eventually carry out 250,000 operations a year on NHS patients – or even, the Secretary of State John Reid (who had replaced Milburn in 2003) speculated early in 2004, up to 15 per cent of the NHS total, or some 640,000 a year.[59] In practice, by early 2004 only two private DTCs had opened. One of the major UK bidders, Mercury Health, withdrew its bid, and in April 2004 the government announced that another of its major 'preferred bidders', Anglo-Canadian, had been 'deselected'. A Department of Health source explained that 'the Anglo-

Canadian deal would have cost ridiculously more than the NHS tariff for these operations'.[60]

The government did not pretend that private providers would contribute new kinds of efficiency that could not be achieved by the NHS in the DTCs it was already running. The idea was simply to introduce private provision to supplement public provision – in relatively standardised, and low-risk, kinds of surgery. But there were larger aims too. At a breakfast meeting in Downing Street in May 2003 Tony Blair told a group of 'private-sector health care executives' and some managers of NHS-run DTCs: '... we are anxious to ensure that this is the start of opening up the whole of the NHS supply system so that we end up with a situation where the state is the enabler, it is the regulator, but it is not always the provider'. The breakfast guests 'got the impression that they were being invited to bid to run DTCs as a means of entering an expanding market for treating NHS patients'.[61]

Like intermediate care and the use of spare surgical capacity in private hospitals, the introduction of privately run DTCs/ITCs was advertised as a means of adding to the total supply of services available. But in September 2003 the government admitted that privately owned DTCs could recruit up to 70 per cent of their staff from the NHS workforce. It turned out that there were no pools of unemployed doctors and theatre nurses in South Africa, Canada, the USA, etc., so an influx of skills from these places had never been on the cards. Instead of bringing substantial new resources, the new privately owned centres would be taking them away from the NHS. Then it emerged that the new centres' guaranteed five-year supply of patients – a guarantee they had insisted on to make their proposed investment profitable – was in some places much more than any excess demand for treatment.[62] In other words, they would be taking away not only staff but also patients who were actually being treated in good time in existing NHS hospitals and surgical units, leaving these with excess capacity and making them suddenly high-cost. In November 2003, for example, the southwest Oxfordshire Primary Care Trust rejected a government-sponsored proposal that it should hand over a large proportion of the cataract operations currently performed by the Radcliffe Infirmary in Oxford to be carried out instead in one of a chain of new ITCs to be run by the South African company Netcare. Two weeks later, however, following heavy pressure from the Department of Health via the local strategic health authority, and a commitment to cover the £250,000 income shortfall that the change would mean for the Radcliffe, the PCT board was induced – by a narrow vote – to change its mind.[63]

Secretary of State Reid denounced NHS critics who pointed out the transparent weaknesses of the official case for DTCs or ITCs. They were concerned for their jobs, he said, not for patients, who would get faster treatment thanks to the new centres.[64] The new centres, he insisted, would 'revolutionise' treatment by specialising entirely in elective surgery, so that there would be no cancellations to make way for urgent cases. But NHS-run DTCs were already doing precisely this.

Reid also had difficulty explaining why the private centres were going to be paid substantially more than the rates laid down in the national 'tariff' or price list (described below, pp. 74–75) according to which NHS providers were paid. It was a 'market forces' factor, he explained, to cover their 'start-up costs'.[65] But most people could readily see that it really represented the private sector's higher costs and the need to return a profit to shareholders. It was impossible to guess how much of the planned annual outlay of £2 billion on the new privately owned DTCs/ITCs was accounted for by these extra costs, but it was hard to see the project as adding to the NHS's resources. It seemed likely to cost the NHS a great deal of money and to destabilise its existing facilities. More than anything it looked like a case of cream-skimming for the private sector.*

The NHS Plan and the Concordat, then, clearly signalled the new direction of policy. But just how far and how fast the government was moving towards a radically different health system, in which the determinant logic from top to bottom was no longer social (let alone egalitarian) but commercial, was still not yet fully apparent. It only

---

* The story of the DTCs took an ironic turn in December 2003 when the Independent Healthcare Association, which had negotiated the Concordat with the government, broke up after two of its major members left, apparently in disgust over the way foreign bidders had been preferred to British companies in the allocation of DTC contracts. Commentators believed that the government had preferred foreign bidders because the Department of Health believed that surgery carried out in private hospitals in Britain cost 40 per cent more than the same operations performed by the NHS (see Helene Mulholland, *Guardian*, 12 December 2003). The IHA was reconstituted as an association to represent only long-term care homes.

became entirely clear with the introduction in 2002–03 of a further innovation, equally in line with the vision sketched by Blair over breakfast with the private health care executives: foundation trusts.

Foundation trusts

Foundation trusts were first foreshadowed in a speech by Alan Milburn in February 2002. No mention of them had been made in the Labour Party's election manifesto of the previous year, nor was any White Paper issued about them, though the legislation providing for them, and the detailed guidance later issued by the Department of Health for trusts applying for foundation status, showed that they had been a long time in preparation. According to Milburn, the idea emanated from NHS chief executives. It was presented as merely formalising the greater freedom which the *NHS Plan* promised for the highest-rated NHS trusts. Yet in reality it represented a drastic further step towards a fully marketised system.

Legislation followed swiftly and was completed in the autumn of 2003.[66] Under it all NHS hospitals, and all PCTs, will eventually be eligible for 'foundation' status. Foundation status will be awarded by an independent regulator. Provided they stay within the terms of the regulator's authorisation, foundation trusts will cease to be subject to control by the Department of Health and its regional arms, the strategic health authorities. They will become 'public benefit corporations', to be run as non-profit but nonetheless commercial concerns. Their assets will cease to belong to the state. They will be free to set their own pay scales, borrow on the private market, enter into contracts with private providers, and determine their own priorities.

They will be subject to some legislative constraints, which the government presented as ensuring that the NHS's founding principles would remain intact. They may not charge fees to NHS patients, and fees from private patients may never constitute a larger share of their revenue than at the time they become foundation trusts. There are no shareholders and so no profits. There are limits on how they may dispose of the assets they have inherited. And there will be boards of governors, a majority elected by members of the public in the local area. Indeed the government represented foundation trusts as a democratic advance.[67]

But the legislative constraints are weak, if not deliberately deceptive, above all because foundation trusts' freedom to enter into contracts with private sector companies means that all the things they are themselves prohibited from doing may be done by these joint ventures. A joint venture can for example charge fees, to constitute whatever proportion of its revenues it wants, and it may – indeed must, if it is a joint venture with a private company – make profits and distribute them to its share-holders. It will also be free to finance private loans out of its NHS revenues. In addition, it seems likely that the proceeds from any assets a foundation trust is allowed to sell will not go to the NHS as a whole, for use where needs are greatest, but will boost the balance sheets of the foundation trust alone.

There is also in reality no provision for local control. How many 'members' there are, and how they are selected from the local population, is provided for in each foundation trust's constitution, approved – without any public consultation – by the regulator. There is no require-ment for the 'members' to be representative of the local population or accountable to them, and in the first ten foundation trusts the total number of 'members', including patients and hospital staff, was less than the three per cent of the local population.[68] The 'members' elect a majority of the governors, and the governors appoint the non-executive directors, who in turn will appoint the chief executive. Non-executive directors may be recalled by the governors, but there the governors' power ends. This aside, the board of directors have unfettered power over trust policy. The resemblance to the way power is concentrated in private companies is not coincidental.

Critics were quick to point out these and many other aspects of this complex change. MPs were particularly concerned that the first hospi-tals to become foundation trusts, being free to set their own pay scales and to borrow money, would drain other hospitals of their best staff, creating huge new inequalities, both between hospital staffs and between the facilities available to patients in adjacent areas. But the inequalities that worried the MPs are not a transitional problem; rather they are inherent in the whole idea. Foundation trusts will become like commercial companies. Their sole responsibility is to provide NHS health services 'effectively, efficiently and economically', i.e. to focus on their balance sheets, not on meeting patient needs. Even the regulator is not explicitly charged with meeting patient needs, as the Secretary of State for Health is under the NHS's founding Act, but only to act 'in a manner consistent with' the general duties of the Secretary of State. Foundation trusts will 'not be required to comply with management and operational guidance from the Department of Health', the Department told parliament, and so will be under no obligation to cooperate in service planning covering regions or even the country.[69] They will have the same ability to block area-wide improvements that impinge on their privileges that teaching hospitals have always tended to have (see Chapter 4). The London Health Link (an association of the now abolished community health councils) pointed out that the problems experienced in establishing 'clinical networks' necessary for a system rationally oriented to health needs were already serious enough:

> For example, neonatal intensive care services are being reviewed at the moment because of a drastic shortage of the right type of cots in the right place. The process of negotiating with individual hospitals whose clinicians do not want to 'lose' their status as high level neonatal intensive care units as a result of the creation of a pan-London system has been arduous and lengthy, before consultation with the public even starts.[70]

When hospitals have foundation status, these kinds of problem seem bound to become worse, if not insuperable. The services available to patients will become a by-product of corporate planning focused on financial viability and growth. Not only will they be uneven between areas, they will be uneven between needs. Unglamorous, complex, costly kinds of care will inevitably lose out. What foundation trust will choose to specialise in mental health, geriatrics, patients with chronic diseases, or refugees' health? Who will provide them with an incentive to do so? The strategic health authorities will have no authority over them, PCTs will lack the necessary power, and it is not the job of the regulator. Who will even know what the health needs of their area are?

From costing expenditure to charging prices: the national tariff

The advent of foundation trusts needs to be seen in conjunction with another, less publicised but crucial change, which alters the way in which NHS providers have to calculate their profit and loss. In today's consumer-driven culture it seems extraordinary that for forty years NHS consultations, investigations and treatments had no price tags. In the NHS's formative years the idea of reducing the health care of a patient to a series of transactions on a balance sheet was seen as ludicrous, one of the mistakes of past medical history. But the absence of a pricing system did not mean that there were not strong financial controls and accountability. Expenditure was accounted for in meticulous detail – detail that is completely absent from the accounts that hospital trusts now publish. The paper trail kept the costs of bureaucracy down but provided genuine financial transparency.

During the mid-1980s, however, politicians and economists began equating the need for transparency with prices and market transactions. It became commonplace to say that doctors and nurses did not understand the costs of care, and to lay the blame for the shortcomings of the NHS at their door: if only they understood the cost of each treatment, this would somehow reduce the costs of care. Pricing resulted from this absurdity.

In practice, health care activities vary enormously, with extremely complex interrelationships between activities. Most people do not present with one easy-to-treat condition and even if they do, the range of expertise and specialised departments that must collaborate in its treatment, from pathology and scans to surgery and drugs and rehabilitation, is huge. But people with diabetes, for example, do not just have a problem with their sugar metabolism; the disease affects many organs so that diabetics have an increased risk of coronary heart disease, high blood pressure, blindness, renal failure, ulcers, and so on. Anyone admitted to hospital is soon aware of how different all the patients on their ward are from each other, and how their range of needs and treatments varies. And yet the idea behind pricing and costing is to try to reduce everything to standardised treatments applied to standard patients. This is the sort of activity the market can relate to.

As we saw earlier, the internal market introduced the costing of an individual 'treatment' on the basis of all the various costs associated with it. The total cost would thus have to include a proportion of the rental income, repairs and maintenance, water and energy, staff time, goods and services bought in – and of course a share of the cost of the new bureaucracy needed to undertake all this work. It is obvious that the allocation of all these 'overheads' to any given treatment is arbitrary, and the problem became worse when the Department of Health set about trying to construct standard 'reference costs' for the entire NHS, with a view to putting pressure on hospitals with costs that were much higher than the average. The available data were notoriously fallible, and the Treasury's approach tended to ignore the wide differences in socio-economic conditions affecting the 'case mix' that commonly lay behind variations in performance.[71] Nothing daunted, in 1998 civil servants started publishing 'reference costs' for a wide range of clinical procedures, based on national averages, as benchmarks for judging performance. Then, in 2003, 'reference costs' were transformed into set prices. Now all services were to be bought and sold at the prices contained in a fixed 'national tariff'. For 15 procedures there was now a fixed price that all hospitals must charge, and for other procedures there was a fixed price for all those performed above the contracted number (and at which the 'purchasers' had to be reimbursed for any contracted procedures not performed). By 2005 all procedures are to be priced in this way.

The implication is that hospitals whose costs for any procedure exceed the national tariff will have to give up doing these procedures, or 'subsidise' them from some other part of their budgets. How local patients are supposed to cope with the potentially drastic consequences of such financially driven service changes or cuts was not explained. Presumably they will 'choose' to be sent to some other hospital, however distant, whose costs are lower. Hospitals that cannot provide a service at the price laid down in the tariff will have to cut their costs or abandon the service to another provider that can. Market pressures will, in theory, lead to the most efficient providers taking over. In reality, a whole jungle of new inequalities in provision seems unavoidable.

Regulating standards

By 2001, even the core of the NHS – its hospital and family medicine services – was being transformed into a network of local corporations – the hospital and primary care trusts, and the private companies entering the new NHS 'mixed economy' – operating in a managed market, increasingly like the privatised public services such as water, telephone, electricity and gas. Foundation hospitals would carry this process further still, operating alongside for-profit providers. In effect, a quasi-monopolistic market was emerging which needed regulating.

The government seems to have only gradually come to see the need for regulation in this way. The initial motive seems to have been a desire to identify poorly performing hospitals and bring their performance up to the level of the rest. Another motive was the wish to strip hospital consultants of their remaining policy-making power and give cost-oriented managers exclusive authority. The fiercely defended principle that doctors' clinical judgement must be respected made it difficult even for hospital chief executives to change the balance of service provision or to curb spending that was wanted by some powerful senior consultants. But a series of medical scandals centred around individual doctors, from the Bristol neonatal surgeons James Wisheart and Janardan Dhasmana to the Kent gynaecologist Rodney Ledward, and the case of the serial killer Dr Harold Shipman, helped turn public opinion against the authority of doctors generally, and made it possible to try to introduce more binding guidelines on clinical practice.

'National Service Frameworks', which outlined protocols and service arrangements for improving the treatment of a series of specified conditions including diabetes, coronary heart disease, and mental health, were one means of control. Another was the creation in 2000 of a well-funded Commission for Health Improvement (CHI), to undertake 'clinical governance' reviews in hospitals across the NHS. By early 2002 it had more than 300 full-time staff plus a pool of 500 part-time staff from which teams were drawn to carry out the reviews. A National Institute for Clinical Excellence (NICE), with an initial budget of £9 million, was set up for England and Wales, with a counterpart in Scotland, to assess the effectiveness of drugs and other medical technologies. A large part of its aim was to try to limit the growth of the NHS drugs bill by submitting the sales-oriented claims of the pharmaceutical companies to independent and objective assessment. It also wanted to limit the 'postcode rationing' of new drug therapies by substituting authoritative national judgements about them for the decisions of individual physicians.

None of the elements in this rather haphazard structure proved initially very effective. NICE appeared to be quickly 'captured' by the pharmaceutical industry, which was in any case represented on NICE's governing body. NICE's first attempt to discourage the use of a drug, Relenza, which its expert assessors found to have too little therapeutic benefit, was reversed, and NICE also shied away from evaluating the cost-effectiveness of drugs it did approve.[72] CHI also proved ineffectual. This was partly because of the impossibility of applying standard criteria to hospitals with differing specialties and scales of operation, and partly because the CHI review teams – who were inevitably often less qualified and less experienced than the hospital staff they were inspecting – possessed no magic solutions to the often complex and intractable problems affecting the performance of cash-starved hospital staff. Unless CHI inspectors discovered gross incompetence or negligence there were severe limits to how far their reports could hope to improve anything.[73]

In May 2002 the government moved to improve this state of affairs by creating a single new body, to be called the Commission for Health Audit and Inspection (CHAI), which would combine the work of CHI with the work already done on the NHS by the Audit Commission. CHAI would also take over the work of the National Care Standards Commission which had recently been established to regulate private health care (since, under the Concordat, private nursing homes and hospitals would increasingly be treating NHS patients), and there would be a parallel new Commission for Social Care Inspection. CHAI was intended to become more like Ofsted, 'a single rigorous inspectorate armed with the ability to expose poor practice and highlight good practice'.[74]

At the time of writing it was too early to tell whether standards in hospitals were really likely to be significantly improved by CHAI, or spending on drugs made more rational by NICE. But the creation in 2003 of an independent regulator to license foundation trusts was another matter. As we noted earlier, the regulator will decide what services each foundation trust provides, but will not have the obligation laid on the Secretary of State for Health to provide equal and comprehensive health services for all, and will not be answerable to the Secretary of State, even though he will formally report to him. In practice, the independent regulators of other public service sectors, like the railways and energy, have pursued market-efficiency goals without regard to social needs. For example the rail regulator has cut rail services, lifted the cap on charges for off-peak inter-city travel, and shifted resources away from rural services, while the energy regulator has ended the cap on electricity charges to poor consumers on pre-payment meters. As more and more hospital trusts get foundation status NHS hospital services are liable to be regulated on similar market-oriented lines, with the government disempowered from intervening to ensure the meeting of health care needs, or any other desirable public health goal.

THE EMERGING NHS LANDSCAPE

The transformation of something as big and complex the NHS can only be summarised, in the way this chapter has tried to do, at the cost of many simplifications and omissions. Even so it can be hard to see the overall picture, especially since so many of the changes are still in process while others, like foundation trusts, are just beginning. It is especially hard to distinguish between changes that are welcome in themselves, and those that are not. For example everyone benefits from medical advances, such as less intrusive 'keyhole surgery', that allow people to be discharged much sooner, or even to have 'day surgery' and go home afterwards. On the other hand they do not benefit if the reason for early discharge is financial, not clinical, and leads to suffering, and costly re-admissions. Likewise, with much more money going into the system from 2000 onwards, real improvements are being made; but if this money is diverted to pay for more expensive privately provided plant, like PFI hospitals, or more expensive private services, like those to be provided by for-profit DTCs or ITCs, it is highly undesirable. It is not easy to disentangle changes that are science-driven and rational from those that are ideology-driven and irrational.

One way to see the new shape of things is to relate changes to the NHS's founding principles of comprehensiveness, universality and equity. Comprehensiveness has clearly been abandoned, whether explic-itly, as with most long-term residential care and routine optical care, or implicitly, as with dentistry, which has become available on NHS terms only to children and adults fortunate enough to live near a dentist still willing to work at NHS rates. Universality has gone in as much as the services provided both by GPs and by hospitals vary increasingly from place to place. The push to rectify the unequal geographical distribution of resources, such as GPs and hospital beds, has been largely abandoned too. The emphasis is now on 'decentralisation' and 'choice', but there are no mechanisms for providing democratic local control. If you need a heart bypass operation, your chances of getting one in good time still vary widely according to where you live, and the emerging foundation trust system offers no mechanism for remedying this.

As for equal access in the sense of access based on need, not income, this has been steadily eroded both through the abandonment of comprehensiveness – so that many quite poor people now have to pay as much as the affluent for long-term care, optical care, domiciliary services, etc. – and through charges ('co-payments', in the language of the World Bank) for prescriptions, dentistry, and non-clinical hospital services (such as phones and television). It has also become routine for patients needing elective surgery, such as cataracts or hip replacements, to be told at the hospital what the waiting time is, and then asked if they would like to have the surgery done much sooner, privately. Access to primary care is improving, and should improve still further as more funds reach general practices and specialist clinics of various kinds, more GPs are appointed, and nights and weekends are better covered – improvements that should make hospital accident and emergency facilities less burdened. If this happens the private primary care services that the private health care industry is promoting ('walk-in' clinics and insurance policies for primary care) should not be needed. Otherwise inequity will start to become familiar in primary care too. More problematic is the break-up of continuity in primary care that is implied in the sharing out of primary care services among a range of new providers, including private providers, described in Chapter 5.

Harder to see are the effects of the marketisation of NHS hospitals, and the penetration of NHS hospital services by private industry. The now-required focus on the bottom line already means that profitable services get priority, while costly services such as mental health are as far as possible cut back. Some of the signs are all too clear, even if the root cause is usually officially denied – new PFI hospital buildings with too few beds and too few staff to cope with demand; outsourced meals too unappetising to eat; substandard cleaning or sterilisation of equipment by underpaid outsourced workers, contributing to the rise in dangerous infections; medical accidents due to faulty work by private pathology labs.

At a deeper level still are the implications of the so-called mixed economy of health care. Quite apart from some £4 billion a year of tax revenues going to the private long-term care industry, more and more of the NHS budget itself now ends up in the accounts of private companies providing everything from weekend GP cover and GP premises to surgery in private hospitals. Not only do these services tend to cost more, as the case of the DTCs brought to everyone's attention, but they also tend to destabilise the finances and organisation of NHS hospitals and other services, and so raise their costs too.

With each new insertion of private provision into the NHS the political clout of the private providers increases, and the dominant culture shifts still further in a private enterprise direction, while the structures of national control are being progressively dismantled. Once most if not all NHS hospitals have foundation status, and share the 'market' for hospital care with a wide range of private hospitals in a 'mixed economy of health care', the only remaining mechanism of coordination will be the independent regulator, whose mandate says nothing about comprehensiveness, universality or equity.

By the time most hospital trusts have foundation status and are free to function increasingly like private corporations, unsupervised by the strategic health authorities, this shift in the power balance seems bound to become even more significant. The most expensive part of the NHS – the hospital sector – will then be in the hands of chief executives dealing constantly with a growing system of private providers within and around the hospitals they are operating. It does not follow that they will absorb the ambient corporate culture and start awarding themselves higher salaries, and restructuring hospital services on more and more market-oriented lines. But it takes a lot of optimism not to believe that this is a rather likely outcome, especially in the foreseeable context of the eventual return of a Conservative government pledged to push the privatisation of health services further still.

4

HOSPITALS

At the heart of the NHS, accounting for around two-thirds of all spending, is the publicly-owned system of hospitals.[1] Patients and their families are always grateful for the care these hospitals provide, but this feeling is often mixed with reservations about quality – poor food, poor levels of cleaning, decaying or neglected fabric (it is still not uncommon to find wards housed in portacabins or temporary structures that have gradually become permanent), delays, too few and too busy staff – and an environment that too often feels difficult or even hostile when it should be sympathetic and caring. Doctors, too, complain of being ashamed of the buildings they work in and their of lack of access to equipment and high-quality facilities, compared to their European colleagues. But while many of these problems clearly stem from inherited weaknesses and underfunding, others are due to changes that have occurred since the early days of the NHS – above all, higher patient expectations, the shorter average length of stay, loss of continuity in care, and new levels of shortages – especially of staff and beds.

Some of these changes are due to medical advances that have altered the tempo and complexity of hospital life in all advanced economies. Powerful new diagnostic technologies and therapies allow for shorter stays in hospital and for more care to be provided outside hospital – yet they also involve more specialisation, more tests, more possibilities for breakdowns in communication, with patients shunted between departments for CAT scans, blood tests, ultrasounds, and the rest.

Figure 4.1 The distribution of total NHS spending in England, 2002–03

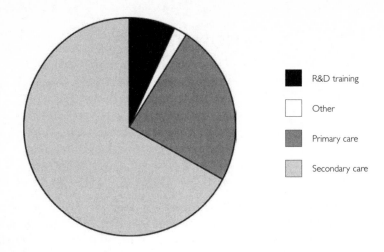

Source: Department of Health, *Delivering the NHS Plan – expenditure report*, London, April 2003

But what lies at the heart of the most distressing problems experienced by both patients and staff is not scientific and technical change but the application of a new business model and business culture to hospital management. It is the business model that has squeezed out low-tech but essential care, including rehabilitation and preventative services such as speech and language therapy, physiotherapy, chiropody and dietetics, which in some places people can only get by 'going private'. It is the business model that underlies the drive for 'efficiency savings' and 'performance targets', such as higher 'throughput', leaving fewer nurses and staff looking after more patients with greater levels of health care needs. It is the business model that makes NHS 'bed managers' behave, against their will, like bailiffs acting for a ruthless landlord, eager to evict one set of patients to make room for another (the existing patients have used up their quota of care, the next patients bring new cash). Lack of bed capacity, and pressure for the earliest possible discharge, see patients moved from ward to ward, or marooned in remote parts of the hospital. There is even a label – 'medical outliers' – for these orphans of the system, while those who can't be evicted soon enough to make room for new patients are known as 'delayed discharges', or 'bed blockers' – second-class citizens cluttering up the wards. As hospitals compete for trade, they trade away care and humanity.

Proponents of the new business model often try to justify it in terms of medical progress. A high turnover of patients is said to be a rational consequence of improved diagnosis and treatment, while improved diagnosis and treatment, and the higher expectations these give rise to, are seen as constantly driving up costs, necessitating a more 'businesslike' approach to hospital care. But the real driving force behind the business model, as we have seen in Chapter 3, is political and ideological. As Table 4.1 (on the following page) shows, the US evidence suggests that business-oriented medicine in fact performs less well, spends more on administration, and costs more per patient overall.[2]

Adopting the business model also means abandoning hospital planning for the nation as a whole, by means of which the NHS was once gradually moving towards the goal of universal and equal health care. That planning model is criticised today as outmoded, involving 'command and control', and 'one-size-fits-all standardisation', as opposed to the business model which is supposed to offer 'choice'. Yet it is precisely the model of hospitals as so many business units, competing to supply standardised products to standardised 'consumers', that underlies the dehumanisation and stress experienced by patients and staff today. The new business model is in fact a regressive reaction, exploiting shortcomings that were, to a very large extent, inherited from the pre-NHS years.

THE INHERITED HOSPITAL SYSTEM AND THE NHS RESPONSE

On 5 July 1948 the NHS inherited some 2,700 hospitals in England and Wales with a total of 480,000 beds, and 417 hospitals in Scotland with some 64,000 beds.[3] Despite the scale of this inheritance, it was a poor one. Around 45 per cent of hospitals in England and Wales had originally been built before 1891, and 21 per cent before 1861. Add to this

Table 4.1 Clinical performance and cost efficiency in US for-profit and non-profit health maintenance organisations, and for-profit and public hospitals, 1994

Clinical indicators	Percentage of eligible patients receiving interventions	
	For-profit HMOs	*Non-profit HMOs*
Beta-blocker after myocardial infarction	59.2	70.6
Annual eye examination for diabetics	35.1	47.9
Complete immunisations	63.9	72.3
Mammography	69.4	75.1
Cervical cytology	69.4	77.1
Cost efficiency indicators	*For-profit hospitals*	*Public hospitals*
Administration as share of total costs, 1994 (%)	34.0	24.5
Rise in administration costs 1990–94 (%)	2.2	1.2
Cost per patient at discharge from hospital, 1994	$8,115	$6,507

Note: All cost efficiency data controlled for hospital type, case mix, and proportion of revenues from outpatients, census region and local wage levels

Source: D. Himmelstein and others, 'Quality of care in investor-owned vs not-for-profit HMOs', *Journal of the American Medical Association* 282, 1999, pp. 159–63; and S. Woolhandler and D. Himmelstein, 'Costs of care and administration at for-profit and other hospitals in the United States', *New England Journal of Medicine* 336, 1999, pp. 769–74

the six years of bomb damage during the Second World War, plus arrears of repairs and maintenance, and the hospital system was a sorry picture. The official historian of the NHS, Charles Webster, called it a 'ramshackle and largely bankrupt edifice'.[4]

In 1948, prior to the creation of the NHS, charges for treatment in the so-called voluntary hospitals, where most acute care was provided, were two and a half times their pre-war levels, yet still woefully inadequate to maintain, let alone improve, hospital buildings and equipment. Poorly paid young consultants – i.e. specialists – struggled to eke out a living by odd teaching jobs, and 'vast tracts of the country were dependent on whatever consultant skills local general practitioners could muster'.[5] The inherited facilities were in desperate need of investment, and still more would be required to change the inherited distribution of resources around the country. Policy-makers were forced to accommodate a range of vested interests, including those of the major teaching hospitals and their boards, which hampered change. Hospital doctors had only been reconciled to becoming salaried employees by being given 'merit awards' to top up their salaries, plus the right to practise private medicine on the side and to look after their private patients in 'paybeds' in NHS hospitals. The major teaching hospitals were also allowed to stay to a significant extent free from direct control by local health authorities.

This was the backdrop against which the architects of the NHS had to devise a system capable of overcoming or at least ameliorating the system's historic flaws. They were well aware of all the problems, but building the capacity to deal with them took time and money. Thus, for example, in 1948 there was little systematic collection of data on inequalities in access to care – the necessary systems and expertise had to be created almost from scratch. Routine statistical data, which were of key importance if hospital resources were to be more equitably distributed, were not systematically collected until 1955 when an NHS statistician was appointed and routine hospital statistical returns were designed.[6] It was a measure of the inertia that had to be overcome that as late as 1956 the authors of an official report had to remind hospitals and regional administrators that a national system was in place: 'Regional Hospital Boards should be told, and hospital Management Committees should accept, that the Regional Boards are responsible for exercising a general oversight and supervision over the administration of the hospital service in their Regions'.[7] Expertise to manage the NHS's 'estate' also had to be developed (a chief architect was appointed only in 1958), along with the capacity to oversee capital investment and ensure the nation-wide surveillance of public health. The teaching and training of medical staff, even though the Royal Colleges were heavily involved, also had to be systematised and integrated with hospital development.

Thus the scale of the required investment in capacity and new skills can hardly be overstated, while progress was always hampered by the Treasury's anxiety to limit costs. But the architects of the NHS showed great ingenuity, and in spite of all the compromises that had to be made, the new systems that began to emerge were a growing success.

Advances in medical science helped too. Epidemics of infectious diseases were on the wane even before the advent of antibiotics, but during the NHS's first decade antibiotics made the large Victorian infectious disease hospitals redundant. Chest physicians, once the kings of huge empires founded on tuberculosis and rheumatic fever, found their services no longer needed and the specialty shrank, overtaken by new specialties including diabetes, coronary heart disease, stroke, cancer and geriatric medicine. At the same time the huge Victorian Gothic institutions that housed the 'insane', the 'mentally retarded', 'incurables' and 'older people' were made redundant by changing public and medical attitudes and new treatments. Medical practice changed in other ways too. Improved medical knowledge meant that people who had suffered heart attacks, once deemed to require prolonged periods of bed rest, were now subject to early discharge and rapid rehabilitation. People with complex chronic conditions, from diabetes to mental illness, were now no longer primarily looked after in hospitals but were cared for by their GPs. Advances in drug therapy, vaccination, immunisation and diagnostic capabilities, as well as in surgery and medical technology, all contributed to earlier diagnosis, new ways of working and a substantial growth in community-based care. Day surgery, laser therapy and micro-invasive techniques such as angiography and angioplasty also transformed the time needed in hospital for many groups of patients.

On the other hand, with many more sophisticated treatments becoming available the tempo of hospital life became more rapid, and organising it became more complicated. Higher public expectations led to the phasing out of many of the old 'Nightingale' wards with twenty or thirty beds, while tight restraint on NHS expenditure held down salaries, leading to a big increase in reliance on nurses and doctors from abroad, and on agency staff; and to the end of the old strict hierarchical discipline of nurses under fearsome matrons. Financial cutbacks also led to the diminution and, eventually, virtual elimination of NHS hospital care for the chronically ill. Respite care for people with chronic illnesses or with devastating diseases such as motor neurone disease or Parkinson's disease is no longer provided in hospital – or indeed anywhere in the NHS; patients and carers now struggle on with often minimal medical support and intervention. Financial pressures have often resulted in the closing of day rooms, leaving no tranquil space for patients and visitors, and no rooms where staff can comfort distressed relatives. The frantic atmosphere depicted in *Holby City* is quite typical of the acute hospital today.

Through all such changes, however, from 1948 to 1980 the NHS's founding goals of universality, comprehensiveness and equity were doggedly pursued, and the legacy of inequality from the pre-war years was gradually reduced, in spite of constant pressure from the Treasury to limit spending (indeed in some years there was an almost complete ban on new public investment). But from 1980 onwards, the Treasury's focus on cost containment turned to market solutions. The vested interests in the inherited hospital system which had been kept at bay for three decades gradually returned to power, and the progressive institutions that had been set up to contain them were dismantled. To understand this process we need to take a brief look at what these interests were and how they were incorporated into the NHS.

ACUTE HOSPITALS

The acute hospital of today has its origins in what used to be called the 'voluntary' hospitals where, before 1948, honorary consultants provided the bulk of the nation's specialist inpatient care. The voluntary hospital was a charitable institution where doctors often treated the poor for little or no charge, and the gentry for substantial fees. This remained the dominant model even after the rise of the municipal hospitals in the 1920s, with a higher share of the total number of beds.[8] When a hospital patient no longer needed a hospital consultant's services he or she was either sent home, with some sort of domiciliary services arranged for, or transferred to a ward for the chronically sick – usually an NHS geriatric ward – in one of the municipally run ex-workhouse hospitals. In 1975 the legacy was still clearly visible: 'In most larger towns', a contemporary hospital doctor observed, 'there will be an ex-voluntary hospital, possibly dating from the early twentieth century, extended and partially renovated piecemeal. The other major institution is likely to be an ex-workhouse of older vintage and drearier aspect'.[9]

TEACHING HOSPITALS

Among the former voluntary hospitals the NHS teaching hospitals, where doctors and nurses were trained, were pre-eminent. Located in London and the major provincial cities, they were exempted from the administrative structure of the new regional hospital boards and were answerable directly to the Minister of Health. They were allowed to retain their independent boards of governors, the right to select patients, and their often-valuable endowments. While for most voluntary hospitals all that was really nationalised was their overdrafts, the teaching hospitals' boards, filled with the great and the good, were allowed to retain their charitable funding, which gave them a useful surplus for both capital and revenue purposes. In particular it became common for teaching hospitals to use charitable funding for capital investment while relying on the NHS for the necessary running costs, making the pattern of funding still more unequal. And while it is doubtful whether the private beds the teaching hospitals were allowed to retain ever made a profit, the impression they gave of extra resources, combined with opportunities for private practice, proved a potent lure for aspiring young consultants. Teaching hospitals associated with university medical schools had prestige and a cachet which, combined with better resources, allowed them to attract better and more staff and still further resources, which in turn enabled them to influence NHS policy more generally.

In the early 1950s it cost twice as much to maintain an inpatient in a London teaching hospital as in an ordinary provincial hospital.[10] Teaching hospitals also enjoyed a conspicuous salary advantage under the system of special distinction awards for senior clinicians. In March 1949, a consultant appointed at age thirty-two could expect a final salary of £2,750; in the same year the top distinction award (received by 4 per cent of consultants) was worth an additional £2,500, or almost as much again.[11] (In 2003 the two figures were £70,715 and £67,079 respectively).[12] London was especially privileged in this respect. In 1949 the consultants in a single London teaching hospital, Guy's, were in receipt of as many 'A' merit awards as all the consultants in the Newcastle, Leeds and Sheffield regions put together.[13] Moreover many teaching hospitals were effectively groups of hospitals, which gave them additional influence. For example, St Thomas's in London also included the Royal Waterloo Hospital for Children and Women, the General Lying-in Hospital, and the Grosvenor Hospital for Women. This pattern continues today.

Teaching hospitals thus continued to be powerful forces in the determination of where NHS revenue went. It was not until 1974, at the height of a government expenditure crisis, that a Conservative Secretary of State for Health, Sir Keith Joseph, stripped teaching hospitals of their boards and made them directly accountable to health authorities.[14] This change, combined with restrictions on paybeds and private practice, placed a check on the investment decisions of teaching hospitals and limited some of their scope for heavy political lobbying.

But in the 1980s these restrictions began to be lifted again and teaching hospitals resumed their influential position, too often at the expense of other sectors of the NHS. In 1994, for example, London's Guy's Hospital was allowed to plan an extension which would be paid for by £13.2 million coming from charities, including £5 million from the carpet magnate Philip Harris (later Lord Harris and deputy chairman of the Conservative Party), with most of the remaining £17 million provided by the NHS. The project ran into problems and at a late stage Harris withdrew half his donation, leaving the NHS to pick up the tab, with a resulting loss of capital by other hospitals and services in the region.[15] Of course this distortion of capital distribution also had considerable revenue implications, diverting revenue away from other services.

Another example concerns health services for children. In 2000 Camden and Islington health authority, together with the medical director at the local University College London Hospital Trust, suggested that the time had come to integrate all the paediatric services across the three hospitals in the area so as to provide continuity of care for all local children. But the Great Ormond Street Hospital for Sick Children was unwilling to go along with this proposal. Nothing fills the collection cans faster than the spectacle of a sick child, especially a child with cancer. Great Ormond Street also had a particularly rich endowment (partly thanks to the playwright and novelist J. M. Barrie, who left it the copyright to his *Peter Pan*) and was about to rebuild its entire plant with funds raised by appeals. It didn't need government capital funding and was in a powerful position to put its own priorities before patient needs or planning. The debate was silenced. Plans for an area-wide children's services strategy are still unresolved. Many other examples could be given.

Teaching hospitals were the chief beneficiaries of Bevan's other concession to hospital consultants, permitting 1.3 per cent of hospital beds to be set aside for consultants' fee-paying patients. In 1975 the Labour Minister of Health, Barbara Castle, proposed ending this arrangement, and in 1976 1,000 paybeds were phased out. The remainder were scheduled to be withdrawn at six-monthly intervals.[16] There was a great deal of resistance to this decision and one of the first acts of Margaret Thatcher's government in 1980 was to reverse it. The Thatcher government also revised the NHS consultants' contract, allowing all consultants – not just those on part-time contracts – to do private work without any significant loss of salary. But where Bevan's concession over paybeds had been made in order to secure the consultants' participation in the new, free, health care system, by the 1980s paybeds were justified as income earners for hospitals. In 1982 a minister even suggested that paybeds should be introduced in cottage hospitals 'so that these establishments can be preserved'.[17] Most NHS paybeds were in teaching hospitals, giving them yet another financial advantage.

HOSPITAL DEVELOPMENT: FROM PLANNING TO THE PFI

The NHS grew out of a consensus about the need for equal access for equal need, which also led to a consensus about the need for planning. A truly national health service implies a comprehensive approach to health care, focused on population needs.

To Enoch Powell, a Conservative health minister, belongs the credit for having provided the political inspiration behind the first coherent national plan for hospital building. His 1962 Hospital Plan has been described as 'a first, normative attempt to alter the distribution [of resources] through a system of capital planning for new hospitals based on the idea of levelling up the standards of service to achieve bed:population norms'.[18] The plan involved the construction of 90 new general hospitals and the remodelling of another 134. Powell also extracted from the Treasury a promise that there would be capital spending in each financial year, something the NHS had seldom enjoyed.[19] Indeed between 1948 and 1962 only £157 million had been spent on capital projects in the whole of the NHS. But the 1962 plan was about much more than hospital building: it also involved investment in primary and community health services. Powell's priorities embraced disadvantaged groups as well as disadvantaged areas: he wanted the principal beneficiaries to be the elderly, the mentally disturbed and mothers with young children.[20] Thus the plan was about redistribution within the three sectors of the service – the hospital service, the family doctor service, and a community-based nursing service with public health functions – as well as between regions of the country. As Powell himself noted at the time, this was 'planning on a scale not possible anywhere else, certainly this side of the iron curtain'.[21]

Powell's hospital plan established district general hospitals (DGHs) – general hospitals of 600–800 beds, serving populations of 100,000–150,000, which by 1991–92 would be carrying out 90 per cent of all acute hospital activity.[22] On the other hand it also met the Treasury's requirement that the capital programme should not lead to an increase in hospital running costs; it envisaged 'a substantial reduction in total [bed numbers] and opportunities for economies from fewer centres and more efficient newer buildings'.[23] Since running costs were thought to increase by £150,000 for every £1 million of capital spending, the plan's investment programme of roughly £1,000 million over ten years implied an annual increase in running costs of £150 million. The plan claimed, however, that the NHS's running costs (£932 million in 1962) would be reduced, not increased.[24] But that could only be achieved by hospital closures, and in fact 1,250 smaller hospitals were closed by 1975.

The Treasury's requirement that the new investment must be justified by demonstrating that it would yield lower day-to-day costs is commonplace in business investment appraisal, and it had been a general objective of the Treasury from the late 1950s. But its adoption for the NHS was a new and significant departure. It was to be a recurring theme from then onwards, and the assumption that new investment would release new efficiencies through service 'reconfiguration' and 'process re-engineering' became enshrined in the planning of all new hospital schemes – and especially of the PFI hospital schemes initiated from the late 1990s onwards.

Investment was a slow process, however, and depended on a continuous growth in NHS funding. NHS Funding did grow through the 1960s, but fell off again in the early 1970s. In the event the plan as originally conceived was never completed, and ten years later many hospitals that were relics of the nineteenth-century Poor Laws were still standing. Of the 224 planned new DGHs only 40 were built, and 'virtually no investment had taken place in modernising facilities for the mentally ill'.[25] Systematic redistribution of both the kinds sought by Powell – i.e. between regions and between groups of patients – had stalled, and by the mid-1970s all public capital investment had entered a long-term decline. Eventually, in 1997–99, there was negative capital investment in hospital and community health services – in those years, more assets were sold or used up than were built (see Figure 4.2).[26] Capital investment would subsequently revive a little, but even so it remained at historically very low levels.

This led to attempts to find sources of capital for hospitals other than government borrowing. From 1973 onwards regional health authorities were allowed to use the proceeds from selling land attached to NHS buildings. Such sales gradually became an important source of funds for capital investment. In 1990 responsibility for capital financing was transferred from the Department of Health to the new 'hospital trusts', modelled on private companies. By 1996/97 the bulk of capital

Figure 4.2 Sources of funding for hospital and community health services (HCHS) capital expenditure, 1986–87 to 1998–99

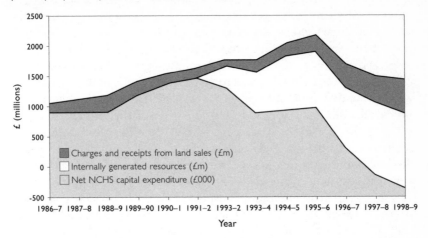

Source: Declan Gaffney *et al.*, 'NHS capital expenditure and the private finance initiative – expansion or contraction?' *British Medical Journal* 1999; 319: 48–51

Figure 4.3 Average number of general and acute NHS beds available daily, England, 1974–2002/03

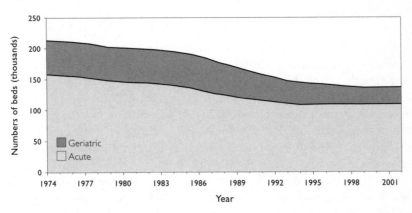

Source: DHSS and DH statistical bulletins 5/85, 1995/20, 1997/20 and 1998/31 and KH03 1998/99–2002/03 (Graph by Alison MacFarlane)

expenditure on NHS hospitals was being financed out of hospitals' revenue budgets or borrowing instead of central government grants. To be able to invest in new equipment or buildings hospital trusts now had either to generate additional income to meet the new debt burden or else make savings elsewhere. Activities such as increasing the numbers of 'paybeds' and renting out hospital forecourts as shopping malls and hospital car parks to NCP became commonplace. The problem was affordability: once capital ceased to be provided free by the government, hospitals undertaking new investment were faced with increasingly difficult decisions about how to pay for it out of their annual budgets.

Since for most hospitals commercial income was limited, the emphasis fell on savings in clinical care. Bed closures and theatre closures, both temporary and permanent, were the only way to cut the principal cost in all hospitals – staff salaries – and this reality dramatically accelerated the process of hospital closures that had begun under the Powell plan. Between 1990 and 1994 245 hospitals were closed in England and Wales, about 10 per cent of the number inherited by the NHS in 1948.[27] Some of the reduction was the result of advances in medical practice, such as day surgery, and some was due to ending NHS provision of long-term care; but a large part of the reduction, which accelerated sharply in the early 1990s, was caused by financial pressures. By 1995 the UK had 4.5 beds per 1,000 of the population, one of the lowest proportions in Europe, achieved by one of the fastest rates of hospital closure in Europe (see Figure 4.3).

Because these later closures were largely unrelated to need, overshoot was almost inevitable. By 1994 researchers had already shown that the current rate of bed closures would put the system under stress by requiring unsustainably high levels of patient throughput and bed occupancy, based on health economists' highly unrealistic expectations about the inexhaustibility of the 'efficiencies' to be wrung from the NHS – and so it proved.[28] Bed shortages were already causing problems in Newcastle upon Tyne, Liverpool, and Birmingham. By the end of the 1990s, in many cities the problems had become crises. 'Efficiency' savings had finally led to many acute hospitals being unable to meet any reasonable definition of demand. Yet further hospital 'downsizing' – the term used to rationalise cutbacks in business – was a central feature of the new wave of hospital investment implemented by New Labour after 1997.

In 1992 the Conservative government unveiled the Private Finance Initiative, described in Chapter 3, whereby the private sector raises the finance for capital investment and receives the contract or lease to design, build and operate new hospital buildings and equipment. The PFI contract, which is usually for thirty years, involves the NHS hospital trust paying an annual charge, which includes payments for the cost of capital and construction, debt servicing and the provision of services such as maintenance and cleaning. Because the costs of privately financed hospitals are relatively high, in consequence of the private sector's higher cost of borrowing and the need to pay dividends to shareholders, hospital trusts embarking on PFI projects found they had to settle for smaller hospitals. Not only were hospitals now reliant on loans instead of grants, they were also forced to raise loans by the most expensive route, from the private sector, instead of through much cheaper government borrowing. In most cases two or even three hospitals would be closed in order to release land and assets to part-fund one new one. The result was an average reduction of 30 per cent in the number of beds and a 25 per cent reduction in budgets for clinical staff during the five-year period between the signing of the contract and the opening of the new PFI hospital; thus the level of services available to patients was being cut, while at the same time NHS assets were being replaced by privately owned ones.[29]

In 1998, in response to mounting clinical and public concern over bed reductions, the Health Secretary, Frank Dobson, set up a national beds inquiry. The inquiry found that further bed reductions associated with PFI schemes could not safely be attained unless alternative forms of institutional provision were put in place.[30] It even recommended an increase in total bed numbers, and government guidance was published calling for a moratorium on NHS bed closures. Despite this, between 1997 and 2002 more than 10,000 NHS beds were closed in England alone.

The national beds inquiry and the *NHS Plan* focused renewed attention on finding substitutes for inpatient beds. A good deal of inpatient clinical care, it was argued, could be provided less expensively in other institutions than acute hospitals. New terms were coined to express this idea, such as 'hospitals without walls', 'hospitals in the community', 'hospital at home', and 'intermediate care'.[31] This approach was usually presented as being underpinned by clinical innovations, or even clinical necessity (for example, staff shortages and new limits to junior hospital doctors' hours of work were given as reasons for hospital service recon-figurations and cuts). But there is considerable evidence that the latest closures were really driven by financial pressures from the PFI and the demand for efficiency savings; in practice, the community-based alter-natives implied in the 'new models of care' rationale for closing hospital beds were seldom if ever provided.[32]

At all events the rate of bed closures was unrealistic, and was a major cause of the problems that have led to so much justified public discon-tent. Demand cannot be met at peak times; emergency admissions take over beds intended for planned surgery; operations are cancelled or postponed; patients wait on trolleys or in corridors; wards and theatres, even whole hospital wings, are temporarily opened or temporarily closed, with patients scattered in inappropriate places.

To pay for the extra debt burden involved in Edinburgh's new PFI-built Royal Infirmary, for example, a 24 per cent reduction in acute bed numbers was required across the area covered by the Lothian Health Board. An assumption was made that new models of 'care in the community' in the area would increase the hospital's productivity by averting the admission of some patients and making it possible to discharge sooner those who were admitted, thus compensating for the reduced bed capacity of the new PFI building. However, these produc-tivity gains were not achieved, nor was the planned substitute provision in the community put in place. Between 1995/96 and 2000/01 there was a much steeper decline in the number of acute beds and rates of admission across Lothian than in the rest of Scotland – in other words, people in need of hospital care were not getting it.[33]

The Worcester Acute Hospitals NHS Trust announced a new PFI hospital in 1996 in the hope that service rationalisation and new effi-ciencies would save it money. But the cost of the new hospital escalated from £49 million in 1996 to £108 million in 1999, mostly because of the extra costs of private finance compared with public borrowing, and the trust's financial problems multiplied.[34] In 1998 the local health authority undertook a strategic review of acute services in an attempt to find extra money to bail Worcester out. Their proposals involved axing one of the area's three district general hospitals, in Kidderminster; cutting bed numbers in a second; and giving a local private hospital an enhanced role in providing services under the NHS. Residents were left with 44 per cent of the beds they had had five years previously, and long distances to travel to get care.

The results were disastrously counter-productive. GPs reported enormous difficulty in getting much-needed hospital care for patients, and even in the summer months the hospitals were on 'red alert' – that is, they were diverting patients to hospitals outside the area. The district auditor's report for 2002 described the Worcester trust as one of the most inefficient in the country because the cuts in clinical resources that were made in order to pay for the PFI meant that consultants were unable to undertake full workloads because no beds were available for admissions.[35] Planned reductions in nursing staff were also based on projected reductions in hospital admissions that turned out be wide of the mark. The trust found itself relying on expensive agency nurses because it did not have enough of its own.

The costs are felt by patients and staff in the loss of the staff levels necessary for adequate, let alone really good, care. Hospitals try to compensate for the loss of beds by pushing patients through faster (faster 'throughput'), to the distress of patients and families. Many hospital consultants now freely admit that whereas NHS hospitals can and often do look after acute emergencies extremely well, care for chronic illnesses and rehabilitation is provided badly or not at all because of the way in which services are being reconfigured and cut.

A vivid picture comes again from Lothian, following a more than usually drastic 'productivity' drive to compensate for too few beds, which occurred well before the PFI.[36] One woman patient described her stay in the Royal Infirmary Edinburgh in 1994 as follows:

The beds never got cold. At times patients are shuffled about like cards in a pack. I was admitted to Accident and Emergency at 3 a.m. By 5 a.m. they had found me a bed in an admission ward, but I was told they were having to discharge patients at that ungodly hour to make room for new admissions. Yesterday two new patients sat in the ward day room from 10.30 a.m. to 5.30 p.m. waiting for their beds to be vacated. Often patients have to be boarded out on any ... ward with an empty bed. Last week an 88-year-old and I were whisked along miles of cold, draughty corridors in three lifts, to spend the night in a gynaecology ward.[37]

In 2003 a retired hospital consultant, Dr Douglas Watt, got a patient's-eye view of hospital care after PFI when he was admitted to Edinburgh's new PFI-built Royal Infirmary following a heart attack. Watt, with forty years' experience working for the NHS, including twenty-eight years as a consultant and seven as a medical director, was horrified by what he found and complained to the Scottish Health Minister, Malcolm Chisholm, that accommodation and services were 'sadly inadequate in almost every aspect' and nursing standards varied 'enormously'.[38] He found poorly ventilated rooms and washing facilities, 'disgusting and inedible food', poor standards of cleaning and hygiene, and high charges for 'amenities' such as television and telephones. Failings in care also appalled this experienced doctor: there was poor continuity of care because of high numbers of agency staff; he had to protect himself from the attentions of an unskilled agency auxiliary who tried to lift him and his various drips onto a commode unassisted; he waited three days to see a dietitian following dangerous pre-operative weight loss, and then saw her too late to do any good. 'During the six post-operative days spent on the cardiac surgical ward, my bed was properly made only three times, with the result that I arrived home with a sacral pressure sore; during my twenty-eight years as a consultant physician, no patient of mine developed a pressure sore de novo whilst under my care'.[39]

Keith Little, a clinical director at the Infirmary, resigned in 1999 because of the shortages, saying: 'In my department [Accident and Emergency] patients are having to wait between two and in the most extreme cases, 10 hours before they can be given a bed'.[40] And a consultant gynaecologist with the Lothian Health Board wrote: 'We work in physical conditions which are not so very different from clinics I have visited in developing countries. ... I know that patients are being discharged from hospital too early or not admitted at all for gynaecological operations because of shortage of beds'.[41] Similar stories are told throughout Britain and are the unambiguous results of hospital downsizing, a signal achievement of the application of market-based thinking to the NHS.

EQUITY IN HOSPITAL FUNDING

In 1948 there were 15.8 consultants per 100,000 people in North East Thames, but only 8.2 per 100,000 in Trent. By 1979 the ratios were 26.5 and 18 per 100,000 respectively, a major improvement, although there was still a long way to go to achieve even a rough equality.[42] Over the UK as a whole, there were other inequalities: for example, some regions did ten times more coronary artery bypass grafting than others. Some patient groups also suffered from unequal provision, for example from inadequate treatment of end-stage renal failure, while conditions for the learning disabled or mentally ill were virtually unimproved.

For a long time progress was hampered by the lack of an agreed mechanism for reallocating resources between hospitals and areas. Funding was allocated on the basis of existing service patterns so that geographical inequalities were reproduced in each year's budget. Attempts to rectify inequalities depended largely on redistributing whatever extra money was put into the NHS each year, but after 1950/51 new money was scarce and almost all the tax revenues allocated to the NHS for capital spending were absorbed by the costs of maintaining the inherited infrastructure. The rational plan that had inspired the originators of the NHS eluded those who had to implement it.

But despite its limited success, Powell's 1962 Hospital Plan kept alive the question of distribution. Politicians were continually reminded of the geographical disparities. In 1969 the Labour Minister of Health, Richard Crossman, complained:

> A terrific lot of money goes into the teaching hospitals, most of which are in the South, and this shifts the balance even more in favour of the London hospitals, with great unfairness to Sheffield, Newcastle and Birmingham, which are really greatly under-financed. The trouble is that the historic costs are gigantic, with about 85% already committed, and I should be very surprised if we could get even 5 per cent reallocated in any one year, especially a year of appalling constriction such as this.[43]

Crossman tried to avoid replicating unequal resource distributions by introducing a population factor into the allocations, but a more systematic approach had to await the Resource Allocation Working Party (RAWP), which was established by another Labour Minister of Health, Barbara Castle, and reported in 1976.[44] The RAWP recommended a payment-per-person formula adjusted according to an indicator of health care needs – standard mortality ratios – to produce a revenue target for each region.[45] The RAWP was criticised on various grounds, especially for using mortality data as a measure of need and omitting data on deprivation.[46] But its chief weakness was its unfortunate timing. Its introduction coincided with a new period of low revenue growth and cash limits on government spending. This meant that equalising resources according to need involved levelling down rather than levelling up. Areas that lost revenue had to cut services – typically cutting long-term care beds and closing hospitals.

A feature of the RAWP with significance for the future was that it introduced a business-oriented approach to capital allocation. The existing capital assets of all NHS hospitals were measured, based on their bed numbers. Short-stay beds were valued at £24,000 each (using 1975 values) and long-stay beds at £12,000, discounted according to the age of the hospital (for example, beds in hospitals built between 1949 and 1961 were valued at 50 per cent of a new bed and beds in pre-1919 hospitals were valued at 30 per cent). The resulting total capital value of all the UK's NHS hospitals was then apportioned to the regions according to a weighted population estimate, to provide capital targets when allocating new resources.[47]

Meanwhile other financial policies were introduced to enhance management's capacity to measure and control hospital costs. By 1979 it had already become conventional wisdom that hospital efficiency depended on the kind of financial accounting used for making economic decisions in market economies, in which costs are related to units of output and policy choices are based on minimising these costs. One change in this direction involved linking costs and clinical activity in order to measure workloads in money terms, using the new concept of 'casemix' in order to estimate what the average cost per inpatient case ought to be. ('Casemix' is a way of making resource allocation fairer by taking account of the range and complexity of the cases admitted to a hospital.) A Royal Commission on the NHS in 1979 said that hospital doctors should become 'explicit resource managers' and recommended that hospitals should be able to keep and spend a proportion of any savings they made, as an incentive to save.[48] But the commission found that hospital financial management was too weak to make this possible. Their own financial adviser told them that 'cost data necessary for planning, decision making and resource allocation are difficult to derive. Important decisions have to be taken with only approximate knowledge of their cost'.[49] The commission concluded: 'it is essential that information on costs must be improved and costed options considered if the best use is to be made of the service's resources'.[50]

MANAGEMENT REFORMS

The obstacles to running hospitals like businesses were finally overcome by the Conservatives' electoral victory of 1979. This changed the political agenda and put in question the assumptions underpinning all public services, including the NHS. The boundary between public and private became increasingly blurred and the focus shifted away from the reduction of social inequality. As we saw in Chapter 3, the NHS was subjected to a severe financial squeeze, while health authorities were obliged to outsource support services and encouraged to purchase care from the private sector. 'Option appraisal', a management technique introduced in 1982, was the discipline for evaluating decisions to 'contract out' to the private sector, and depended on having comparable data for the public as well as the private sectors.[51] Use of this technique increased the pressure to give hospital managers the business management tools and powers they needed.

The answer came in 1983 with Sir Roy Griffith's NHS Management Inquiry. Griffiths recommended a general manager in every hospital and at every level for each tier of the NHS, a major cost improvement programme, and a commercial reorientation of the NHS 'estate' – i.e. its land and buildings. Griffiths wrote:

> The NHS does not have a profit motive, but it is, of course, enormously concerned with control of expenditure. Surprisingly, however, it still lacks any real continuous evaluation of its performance against criteria. Rarely are precise management objectives set; there is little measurement of health

output; clinical evaluation of particular practices is by no means common and economic evaluation of those practices extremely rare.

The immediate need, according to Griffith, was for general managers: 'By general management we mean the responsibility drawn together in one person, at different levels of the organisation, for planning, implementation and control of performance'.[52]

General managers – later chief executives of hospital trusts – replaced 'management by consensus' (i.e. consensus among the senior consultants and administrators in NHS hospitals and health authorities) and created a management structure capable of running hospitals like businesses. Budgetary power was shifted from districts down to hospitals and serious attempts were begun to determine the cost of each clinical activity, holding out the promise of tighter measurement and control of clinicians' work by business managers.

THE 'INTERNAL MARKET'

Until 1990 hospitals were given block budgets, based in principle on plans for meeting the service needs of the local population. Now, however, with the creation of the internal market, hospitals were supposed to compete with each other for contracts from the purchasers (health authorities, GP fundholders and private patients). This meant that a system of pricing had to be introduced, which not only introduced market disciplines into hospital operations but also for the first time enabled the private sector to gain a foothold in the NHS infrastructure.

These developments reflected the growing influence of the US doctrine of applying business principles to health care delivery.[53] By the early nineties the marketisation of health care had become an international trend, and the Department of Health was increasingly drawing its ideas from the international policy arena. Hospital payment mechanisms based on price and contracts were now widely seen as 'incentives for motivating providers' (that is, they were seen as incentives for driving down costs), and throughout the OECD countries a search was under way to identify more effective incentives. The goal was nothing less than 'control over input mix and level, outputs and scope of activities, financial management, clinical and non-clinical administration, strategic management, market strategy and sales'.[54] Service development was now firmly under the control of health economists, not doctors or epidemiologists.

But the execution of this policy depended on another development – the inclusion of a cost of capital in the computation of hospital costs. In order to get hospital managers to manage the hospital's capital assets efficiently the managers were now required to generate a type of profit or return on capital: 'A system of capital charges is an important part of bringing the capital costs of health care explicitly into the minds of health care managers'.[55] Hospitals now had to pay the Treasury an annual charge on the value of their assets and this charge was reflected in the prices they charged purchasers. The rate of interest chosen – the 'capital charge' of 6 per cent – was comparable to a private sector rate of return. Now hospital managers were bound not by national norms for meeting the health needs of their local population but by the requirement to meet increasingly exacting financial goals.

Capital charges also made public and private hospitals comparable in financial accounting and cost terms, which made it easier to contract out services to private providers. Those who wanted the private sector to take over could now argue that it did not matter whether services were provided by the public or the private sector because their costs were now computed on an identical basis. This argument would prove hugely important from 2000 onwards, when the Labour government initiated the opening up of NHS clinical care to private sector providers.

The new quasi-market was 'internal' because at this stage all the players in it were NHS hospitals and community services, but the new trusts were nonetheless based on the principles of local ownership of assets and maximising rates of return on these assets. All the statutory duties imposed on the new trusts were financial. Their principal duty was to earn a specified return. Loose 'mission statements' produced by each trust's board of governors replaced national norms of service provision: for example Dartford and Gravesham hospital trust said it aimed 'to be recognised both locally and nationally for the excellence and ease of access of our services'. Cumberland Infirmary said its mission was 'to provide the best care and highest quality of service to the maximum benefit of patients'. Instead of medical goals, comparative efficiency became the key hospital management watchword.

But few politicians could countenance the closure of acute hospital facilities in their constituencies. This was a particular problem in the Home Counties, where hospitals' capital values were higher and could rapidly undermine their financial viability through correspondingly high capital charges. In Kent, the subsequently disgraced MP Jonathan Aitken used his influence to get a new Accident and Emergency department for his constituency in Thanet, skewing the provision of services in the area (and helping to lead to the proposed closure of the Kent and Canterbury Hospital). Another example concerned the government-commissioned Tomlinson report on hospital bed provision in London, which purported to show that inner-London residents were over-provided with acute hospital beds. Although the report was challenged (especially on the grounds that it failed to take into account the relative absence of other forms of care in London and the relatively high health needs of London's population), the government accepted its findings.[56] But London was part of the government's political heartland and the reduction threatened the possible closure of Guy's and Thomas's Hospital, which served MPs at Westminster. So perhaps it was not surprising that instead of letting 'market rationality' deal with the problem, the government proposed that a reduction of bed numbers should be achieved through a 'firmly managed process' (and Guy's and Thomas's survived).[57] More generally, although the reforms theoretically gave greater autonomy to hospitals, their financial regime remained tightly regulated, so the result was far from being a true competitive market. By the mid-1990s more than two-thirds of hospital trusts' revenues still came from arrangements whereby district health authorities simply paid an agreed amount for a broadly defined range of hospital services over a fixed period of time.

Nonetheless capital charging did lead to hospitals' capital spending being identified as a key part of the cost containment problem: too much was being spent on 'bricks and mortar'.[58] As in business, this encouraged mergers between trusts. In 1997 Paula Mistry estimated in her book *Rationalising Acute Care Services* that hospital cutbacks and trust mergers would eventually reduce trust numbers by about 40 per cent. The reasons she gave are instructive. They were 'increasing market share, cutting overheads … and recognising an inability to continue as a single player'.[59] The language confirms the distance travelled since nationalisation: hospitals were now 'players' in a market, concerned to capture 'market share', minimise costs and maximise surpluses. Clinical practice was progressively subordinated to these imperatives.[60] The 1989 White Paper *Working for Patients* made 'clinical audit' a contractual requirement for hospital doctors and strengthened the hand of hospital managers.[61] It eventually led to the linking of clinical and financial management in new 'clinical directorates'.

THE EFFECTS OF THE INTERNAL MARKET – 'ENTREPRENEURIALISM'

The internal market created a new set of key players, and a new incentive structure, for hospital policy-making. Now the most coveted position was not to be in charge of a regional or district health authority but to be chief executive or director of finance of a hospital – and this in turn could now be a stepping stone to even more powerful positions both within and outside the NHS. Derek Smith, for example, the chief executive of King's College Hospital in south London, went on to become chief executive of London Underground. Hospital chief executives also became more entrepreneurial and had little difficulty in carrying their appointed and generally weak boards of governors with them. The distribution of resources was thus once again uncoupled from the population's need for services, while the restoration of hospital boards of governors ended the direct management of hospitals and services and their local accountability to the local population through district health authorities, and eventually to parliament.

In the new internal market a redistribution of services occurred, but on the basis of financial viability, not the needs of the local population. In the early days of the internal market the chief executive of a mental health trust in London described how local service managers divided up the services and the estate over dinner, rather like properties on a Monopoly board. Horse-trading became commonplace, with chief executives trading services – swapping, say, cancer for gastro services, or head and neck surgery for urology. The aim was to allow each hospital to build up enough expertise to specialise in certain areas, without destabilising the others, but as this was done in the interests of hospitals' financial survival, not patients' needs, it had negative consequences for both patients and clinicians.

The government's focus on particular diseases such as cancer and heart disease exacerbated the problem. New champions such as the cancer and cardiac 'Czars', working together with the pharmaceutical industry, began to create powerful new networks and alliances, and chief executives had to decide how best to position their hospitals in this new and lopsided marketplace. The results often ran counter to good medical practice and holistic, comprehensive care. General surgeons and physicians, for example, need to be able to treat and manage a range of conditions, cases not just of cancer but also of inflammatory bowel disease, ulcers and diverticulitis, etc. Now they found services divided up across hospitals so that they no longer had the mix of cases needed to maintain and develop their skills. A coherent planning framework in which patients' needs were adequately taken into account would have helped to ameliorate or manage some of these conflicts, but the need for hospitals to sustain income by exploiting specialised niche markets won out.

Hospitals, especially the large teaching hospitals, used their charitable funding to try to get a competitive edge and to ensure survival in the internal market. And where the only prospect for financial survival lay in a radical restructuring of the 'estate' they went in for mergers aimed at selling assets and using the proceeds, together with their endowments, to specialise in niche areas. It became common practice for large teaching hospitals to poach specialist staff from neighbouring trusts in order to build up services and compete for patient income. For example University College London Hospital's policy of building up cardiac services involved attracting the two senior cardiologists and their team of some thirty staff from St George's Hospital in Tooting, while the research professor in gynaecological cancer was brought over with fifty staff from Bart's with the promise of several million pounds' worth of infrastructure. (The professor was alleged to have said that it cost UCL and UCLH more to get him than it had cost Real Madrid to sign David Beckham.) There is little public accountability for these decisions. Although responsibility for finding the revenue to finance these commitments remained with the NHS, the local PCTs were not consulted about the major service changes involved and in any case have little power to prevent them.

Another instance of the way in which the internal market led to decisions that were clearly not in the best interests of good medical practice is what happened to the links that had traditionally existed between teaching hospitals and district general hospitals, cottage hospitals and community services. The advantages of such links are numerous. The combined pool of patients and diverse settings provides a valuable base for the clinical training of junior doctors and nurses by exposing them to a wide variety of patients and conditions while allowing standards and quality to be maintained. It isn't always a completely satisfactory arrangement. New consultants and doctors in training are lured to work in less glamorous hospitals by the promise of joint training schemes and split posts with the prestigious teaching hospital, and it would not be unfair to say that sometimes local residents and junior staff lose out when the consultants do not treat both of their split posts as seriously as they should. But when these schemes are operated properly, the advantages can be very considerable, permitting the rational planning of services, taking into account both patients' and staff needs.

A good example was Hackney, an inner-city area in the East End of London with a high birth rate, very high levels of social deprivation, and a large immigrant community. Its local district general hospital, the Homerton Hospital, was a training satellite of St Bartholomew's in Smithfield, while the Queen Elizabeth children's hospital was similarly linked to Great Ormond Street, the major teaching hospital for sick children in London. The Queen Elizabeth (QEH) was a model of how a hospital in a severely deprived inner-city area should be run. Accessible, open and caring, and with exceptional expertise, its junior doctors and nursing staff worked on rotation from Great Ormond Street and many of its consultants had joint appointments with Great Ormond Street. They offered a superb service to needy children and their families.

But in 1991 independent hospital trusts were established; hospitals became consumed with the need to minimise costs, and sought mergers with each other on this basis. The logical merger in this case would have been between QEH and Great Ormond Street, but following its review of London acute hospitals the Tomlinson report recommended that Homerton Hospital should merge with QEH. Great Ormond Street wrote to its consultants saying they must choose which site they wished to remain on, as they could no longer have split posts. At the same time, perhaps understandably, the consultants at QEH wrote a letter saying they would not be prepared to have joint appointments with the Homerton since there were no training links there. In the end the QEH was merged with the Royal London Hospital in Whitechapel – a hospital and community with which QEH had no ties. But then, when faced with a deficit, the Royal London Trust had no qualms about relinquishing the unprofitable side of its concerns, and the poor relation was sold off in order to realise its assets. Thus in 1994 the City and Hackney health authority announced plans to close the QEH in 2003 and to relocate services in the new replacement hospital which was being planned for the Royal London. Then in 1997, for financial reasons, the closure date was brought forward to summer 1998. Residents were not told that the decision was linked to underfunding and the internal market. Despite vigorous opposition from the community health council and local people, the QEH was closed. In 2003 the new hospital was still at the planning stage and children in need of intensive care had to be taken south of the river.

THE RENEWED FOCUS ON PRIVATE PRACTICE

The internal market also turned a new spotlight on the role of private practice in NHS hospitals. Although NHS hospitals were only supposed to treat private patients so long as NHS patients were not adversely affected, this private practice was never contested or challenged by health authorities, despite the fact that waiting lists continued to rise.[62] A report by the House of Commons Health Select Committee in 2002 found there was little benefit in NHS hospitals treating private patients and suggested that the beds should be used for NHS patients instead, but the government did not act on it.[63] The financial pressures on NHS hospital trusts encourage them to turn to private patient income as a means of staying afloat, to the point where the NHS today is actually the largest single provider of private health care through the reservation of 3,000 NHS acute hospital beds – some 3 per cent of the total – as paybeds, 1,300 of them in separate 'private patient units'. In 2002, total NHS income from private patients was £359 million, up 7.6 per cent on the previous year, when more than 1 million people were waiting for treatment at NHS hospitals. The highest private fee earners were NHS teaching hospitals, especially in London, where about one-third of all private patients in NHS hospitals are concentrated.[64] The top earner in 2002 was the Royal Marsden cancer hospital, which received £19.3 million from private patients, representing almost one-quarter of its total income.

These hospitals say they need the money to pay for extra services, but admit they could treat more NHS patients if they did not treat foreign and private patients. The Royal Brompton hospital insists that NHS patients are not disadvantaged by its private work, which raises money to buy new equipment. However, a hospital source told the *Observer*: 'Private patients are booked in first, so if [their treatment] over-runs, NHS patients rather than private patients are cancelled'.[65]

In 1998, out of some 23,000 NHS consultants about 16,000 engaged in private practice.[66] Besides creating a two-tier system inside the NHS, private practice corrodes it in other ways. In practice it is difficult to serve two masters. Some consultants dedicate themselves to the pursuit of private practice at the expense of NHS patients and their colleagues. Evidence collected by the sociologist John Yates suggests that the longest waits for NHS treatment for eye, heart and hip operations tend to occur in places where there are many private beds, that the long-wait specialties are the main private practice specialities and that long waiting lists tend to be associated with surgeons who do a lot of private practice.[67] This means that insufficient surgical resources are provided in the NHS and junior surgeons do much of the operating. Health authorities, however, have seldom challenged this state of affairs, and the internal market gave hospitals even more reason to be silent about it.

Hospital trusts have also turned to the provision of private patient beds as a means of attracting or retaining specialists in 'outlying' areas. Following the closure in 2002 of a local private hospital run by BUPA, the Scarborough and North East Yorkshire hospital trust allocated six beds for private work, together with clinic and operating theatre time. Bob Crawford, the trust's chief executive, said: 'We do not welcome having to venture into the private healthcare sector, but there were serious implications for the NHS patient if we did not do so. Recruitment, retention, and capacity would all have become even more problematic than they already are, and as a consequence it would have become increasingly difficult to provide a full range of NHS services'. John MacFie, a consultant surgeon, said of the closure of the BUPA facilities: 'Those of us with private practices were left in an impossible situation, which the trust has helped to ease'. Senior doctors would have considered moving in search of other private facilities, MacFie said: '… consultants regard their private time as their own and in many cases they use it to support a reasonable lifestyle by treating private patients. Our salaries as consultants are not what they were a decade ago. If the facilities are not available for private work, consultants will look to work elsewhere'.[68]

The *Observer* reported in 2001 that the Department of Health was building private wards for fee-paying patients in various towns where the NHS has become the only provider of private treatment.[69] Hospitals such as Burton General, Hinchingbrook, Luton and Dunstable, St Mary's on the Isle of Wight and Yeovil District Hospital obtained new wards that were the only facilities available for private medical treatment in their areas. Many of Britain's biggest private medical insurers, including PPP, now routinely pay for treatment for customers at NHS hospitals, and indeed some insurers were choosing the NHS as their 'preferred provider', striking deals with chief executives and setting rates accordingly. Some insurers such as AXA SUN even offer patients a cash rebate if they use NHS facilities.

THE SEARCH FOR NEW SOURCES OF INCOME AND 'EFFICIENCIES'

The introduction of the PFI reinforced all the irrationalities of the internal market. New PFI hospitals opening from 1999 onwards discovered that the high costs of servicing PFI debt had landed them with considerable financial deficits – in fact many of the new hospitals were virtually bankrupt before they were even opened. This led them to intensify the search for revenue, competing for both NHS and commercial income and cutting services when no other income could be found.

Events on occasion echoed the closures and service cuts which took place under the internal market. The new PFI hospital in Durham, for example, had to open without its complement of staff and the chief executive of the health authority appealed unsuccessfully for money to meet the extra costs of PFI. In the case of Norfolk and Norwich Hospital, which saw its planned bed complement fall from 1,600 in its 1991 PFI plan to 800 in the final scheme, the local MP also appealed for extra money. In this case it eventually came through a special subsidy and through extra funds when the government decided to create a new medical school alongside the hospital. In London, the University College London Hospitals Trust knew in advance that it would have financial difficulties and began a special fundraising drive, raising £1.5 million from the Teenage Cancer Trust just to furnish the cancer ward with essential beds and equipment. This kind of fundraising drive was replicated elsewhere.

If the search for new sources of income was one of the two main drivers of hospital policy after 1991, the continuing search for 'efficiencies' was the other. By the late 1980s hospital statistics based on 'finished consultant episodes' (FCEs) had been introduced. Clinical activity could now be costed, albeit crudely, and hospital managers could begin to think in terms of a 'hospital production function' whereby managers controlled both inputs and outputs.[70]

Reform of management was a key element of the almost constant political pressure for economy. Rational planning and advances in medical science had already produced a remarkable transformation in efficiency in the first thirty years of the NHS, but the Conservatives' drive for 'efficiency savings' throughout the public services, including savings of 3 per cent a year in the NHS, led to increased efforts. Between 1981 and 1991, while hospital bed numbers fell dramatically, total annual hospital admissions increased from 5.76 million to 7.2 million. Day case activity doubled from 714,000 to 1,550,000 cases a year, and the number of patients treated per available bed almost doubled too. Hospital staff were 'treating growing numbers of patients in declining numbers of beds'.[71]

Where 'efficiency gains' were driven by innovations in clinical practice, such as day case surgery, there were benefits. The move of care into the community, when adequately provided for, was largely welcomed. But the relentless search for productivity and efficiency in a climate of under-funding meant that hospital trust boards had little time to think about patient care. In one hospital where I worked in the late 1990s, I was struck by how the focus of management board meetings was always on the financial statement. At one two-hour management board session we were asked to choose between cutting hard-boiled eggs and cutlery out of the breakfast menu, and axing a nurse post. On another occasion the chief nurse discussed the need to have staff change bed linen every three days rather than daily, and how to dilute the 'rich skill mix' by substituting untrained staff for nurses (an approach actually adopted in the North Durham trust's PFI project, in which some trained nurses have been replaced by 'ward hostesses').[72] Other ideas included turning away all but emergency admissions from purchasers whose contracted patient care allocation had already been used up.

At the same time clinical staff regularly complained of not being able to be innovative or pioneering, and of becoming increasingly inured to the fact that quality was falling because of the decline in nurse numbers and increased use of outsourcing. Clinical care became a constant struggle. 'Efficiency' savings resulted in hundreds of cuts, weakening the morale of staff and severely impairing the quality of day-to-day work and interaction. Surgical teams would operate without lunch because the theatre no longer provided food. Staff eating areas in the canteen were closed, as were doctors' and nurses' dining rooms, and sharing eating areas with patients' visitors meant that doctors and nurses could no longer talk freely about their work. In several PFI hospitals, including the Royal Infirmary Edinburgh, the local Women's Royal Voluntary Service which used to run tea and coffee stalls for patients and relatives lost their space to the much more expensive and more lucrative Starbucks and McDonald's. Staff now had to pay to use the car park, which had been turned over to 'income generation', with daily charges in excess of £10 a day not uncommon. And the rhythm and pace of hospitals changed noticeably as the focus on early discharge, low staffing levels and the use of agency nurses all took their toll. Shift workers found that the canteen hours no longer covered their night breaks and staff on call would be lucky to find a bag of crisps left in the machine dispensing food.

The hospital ward became a noisy and stressful place, rather than comforting and tranquil. Patients would be asked to bring in towels and sheets, and relatives would bring in food because the quality was so poor. Mutual support between patients was eroded too. Income generation now included charging patients to watch TV, and the communal day rooms, which gave access to free TV and where patients could meet and find mutual support instead of being isolated in the area around their beds, were lost to cost-cutting and income-generating measures.

Staff also became increasingly isolated. Patterns of work changed as the hospital was reconfigured along factory lines, with renewed emphasis on shift working and higher productivity. The European working time directive of 1993 meant a major reconfiguring of working patterns.[73] Junior doctors now did shift work, and at nights they would increasingly find themselves covering unknown patients and wards so that continuity of care was broken.[74] With fewer clinical staff and more work to be done, the camaraderie of the doctors' mess was lost – in fact it is now usually deserted. At the same time the skill mix of nurses on the wards was changed, with an increasing reliance on untrained staff. Moreover low wages, poor working conditions and lack of adequate training plans meant that the NHS increasingly had to fall back on agency staff, further eroding continuity of care. Eventually people become worn down and inured to it all – after all, who can they usefully complain to? Teaching hospital consultants flee to private practice, where they have enough time to spend with patients and where the management treats them with respect.

'SUPERBUGS' AND 'SUPERCHEFS'

Outsourcing has changed relationships inside the hospital, creating a new kind of 'social apartheid'. Outsourced workers on lower pay and worse conditions of employment struggle to meet their supervisors' demands, while working alongside NHS staff with higher pay and status who do not always respect them. Not surprisingly this carries serious risks as cleaning, food service, laundry and sterilisation standards fall. But the periodic dramas of hospital 'superbugs' which hit the headlines have not led to official research into the likely impact on infection rates of increased workloads, or of lower-paid and less-highly-trained cleaning staff with rapid turnover, or of new hospitals' poorly designed ventilation and air-conditioning systems and other consequences of market-driven hospital policy-making. Instead of seeing declining cleanliness and rising infection levels as manifest consequences of trying to run hospitals like businesses, market advocates cite them as evidence of an NHS in need of more, not less, 'market discipline'. The government merely declares that hospital infection is a serious cause of mortality, and even that hospitals are dangerous places, which tends to increase public anxiety and reduce opposition to the continuing drive to discharge patients from hospital even earlier.

Similarly the government's response to public complaints about poor-quality food was not to examine the working conditions of outsourced staff in hospital kitchens, or the way in which companies like Sodexho get food prepared by the 'cook chill' method in factories in France and make profits on low budgets. (Audit Scotland found that in 2001, the cost per patient of food and beverages averaged between £1.25 and £3.00 per day).[75] Instead it announced a 'Better Hospital Food Initiative', bringing in 'TV Super Chef' Jamie Oliver and 'Masterchef' Lloyd Grossman to revamp the menus. Patients were predictably unimpressed, and nurses at Blackburn, Hyndburn and Ribble Valley Health Care NHS trusts were reported as pronouncing the new food to be 'slop'.[76]

CLINICAL AUTONOMY CURTAILED

The development of hospitals as businesses and the constant search for cost-cutting measures naturally created continual conflict between doctors and hospital managers over the control of resources. Managers try to meet their new business targets, while doctors try to improve, or least maintain, the quality of clinical care. Hospital organisation changed. Senior specialists were appointed as 'clinical directors', charged with keeping their colleagues in their specialties within budget, while a medical director worked alongside the hospital's chief executive, taking overall responsibility for all the clinical directorates. In this way doctors were left responsible for clinical care, but were also obliged to stay within the financial limits set by the chief executive. Because money now

followed patients – i.e. patients came through contracts paid for by the
health authorities, or later, PCTs, as 'purchasers' – clinicians found themselves facing new barriers to providing comprehensive care. Hospital
consultants seeing patients in outpatient departments would report that
when they found other medical problems they could no longer refer
patients on to their colleagues in other specialties, or indeed for a second
opinion, but had to refer the patient back to their GP. And for expensive
conditions they also found themselves having to gain 'authorisation to
treat' from the purchasing authority. In 2000 the line between clinical
decision-making and general management was formally breached: chief
executives were now given statutory responsibility for the quality of
clinical care – implying ultimate control over how clinical resources are
allocated.[77]

This reform was introduced during the public inquiry into neonatal-
heart surgery at Bristol Royal Infirmary. The inquiry was chaired by
Professor Ian Kennedy, whose book *The Unmasking of Medicine*,
published nearly twenty years earlier, had criticised doctors for arro-
gance and advocated a shift from a professional ethic, based on doing
the best for the patient, to one based on the most efficient use of
resources – in other words, from the doctor's professional ethic to the
manager's, acting on behalf of the state. This proposition marked a
fundamental shift from the traditional clinical relationship where the
doctor acted as patient's advocate. The Bristol inquiry report included
similar views. The authors found doctors' claims to 'clinical freedom' a
'cultural problem': 'against a background of constrained resources, it
may not always be right for the individual doctor treating a particular
patient to insist on having his or her way, if the price to be paid is to
limit or impair the care available for other patients'.[78] But by whom and
how were decisions to be made that weighed an individual patient's
interests against those of the wider community? And had we really
reached the stage where one person's treatment had to be at the expense
of another's? Neither question was adequately answered. Shortly after
finishing as the chairman of the Bristol inquiry, Professor Kennedy was
appointed to head the Commission for Health Audit and Improvement,
in charge of the league tables and performance monitoring which
would play such a crucial role in developing the mechanisms for privatisation and the new regulatory system of the market.

Public criticism of doctors has had a profound influence on clinical practice in hospitals and on the scope for future reform. Some of the criticism was justified: consultants were not directly accountable to anyone, team working among them was often poor, and some were – and a few still are - downright arrogant. This criticism, plus the Bristol neonatal deaths and other medical disasters, paved the way for the introduction of the new clinical governance institutions described earlier. The criticism also gave new impetus to the introduction of for-profit medicine. The government's pursuit of efficiency through stronger links with the private sector would not have been possible without a major dilution of clinical autonomy. A new consultants' contract in 2003 gave hospital management much greater authority over the work of medical consultants, including the freedom to direct them to work in the private sector as employees of the trust. Ironically enough, from the point of view of many consultants the era of lucrative independent private practice was likely to come to an end as insurers, private health care companies and the government tailored policies to allow greater privatisation of clinical care: the pursuit of profits would involve limiting professional autonomy and controlling the setting of consultants' private practice fees.

While changes such as the introduction of audit and quality standards were overdue, the reforms affecting clinical autonomy were implemented as power was shifting from planning bodies to market providers, and from public to private corporations, in the provision of hospital services, and threaten the hospital doctor's advocacy role. Whereas formerly doctors could and did speak out in the interests of their patients, the new balance of power in hospitals means they increasingly cannot. The government's own policy on whistle-blowing makes it more difficult to bring shortcomings to light because under the 2003 consultants' contract doctors face dismissal if they disclose 'any information of a confidential nature concerning patients, employees, contractors or the confidential business of this organisation'.[79] Doctors are now supposed to report their concerns to management and the hospital press office first. Any attempt to do otherwise is interpreted as corporate disloyalty. And when the interests of profit are in conflict with those of patients, as they frequently are in private medicine, the loss of clinical freedom may well become critical.

PERFORMANCE TARGETS AND 'LEAGUE TABLES'

Much of the stress and distress felt in hospitals by the late 1990s resulted from the Labour government's attempt to produce a sort of 'great leap forward' in efficiency through the publication of performance 'league tables' backed by the threat of 'naming and shaming', and the ultimate weapon of sending in what the press liked to call 'hit teams' to take over the management of 'failing' hospitals. Productivity and efficiency were condensed into 'targets' which were used to whip NHS chief executives into making ever-greater efforts to act like businessmen.

It was soon evident that these targets were corrupting the purposes of care. Chief executives resorted to fiddling the figures, as the Audit Commission discovered.[80] Waiting lists became a political issue, so in some hospitals patients waiting for surgery were asked to let the hospital know in writing when they would be on holiday. The administrators would then remove them from the lists for this period, or even deliberately plan their admission for that period so that when patients phoned to say they could not come in they would be dropped from the waiting list. Other hospitals created new waiting lists – waiting-to-get-on-the-waiting-list lists. Money was diverted into meeting centrally imposed targets and away from dealing with the problems trusts actually faced.

The right-wing media exploited Labour's league tables to denigrate the NHS. Doctor Foster's, the coyly named management consultancy (described further in Chapter 7), worked with Imperial College under contract to the Department of Health, using NHS data to compile hospital mortality league tables or 'death charts' which it then sold to the *Sunday Times*. Any statistician will tell you that most of the data on which the tables are based are unreliable if not positively spurious (and an investigation by *Health Service Journal* in late 2003 showed that in 2002 the 'methodology' on which the Department of Health's own rankings are based was changed at the last minute at the behest of the Secretary of State to protect the three-star ranking of certain 'high-profile' hospitals, including one in the Prime Minister's own constituency).[81] But the statistical community has been silent on the issue and publication in the press gives the tables a sort of legitimacy: they are then cited to name and shame hospitals and frighten patients and doctors alike. No doctor wants to be named 'Dr Death' – and so, with the resources available to them being increasingly limited, they begin to make judgements about who will survive and who will not, and about the cost of taking on those most at risk. If a patient is high-risk, will he or she be a liability?

MOVES TOWARDS HOSPITAL AUTONOMY AND PRIVATE SECTOR PROVISION

By 2000, hospital chief executives worn out by the discontent and anxiety of medical staff, and the constant demands and distortions of the 'targets' and 'league table' culture, sought desperately to find ways of escape. At the same time politicians were looking for ways of diverting attention from the deterioration in the health service that their policies were causing, and for ways to offload its debts and deficits. The culture of targets no longer had much credibility with the public, the professions or indeed politicians. But how was the government going to change course without loss of face and credibility, and at the same time how was it going to continue with its project of privatisation, a project that had required so much central control? The answer was to 'devolve' responsibility to hospital trusts and establish a so-called 'mixed economy of care' – i.e. to let for-profit companies provide clinical care, paid for out of tax revenues. This policy, sometimes euphemistically known as 'decentralisation', has become increasingly popular throughout the world in the past twenty years.[82]

In the UK, policy advisers sought advice from the chief executives of the trusts, among which the teaching hospitals were now again in the ascendancy. In 2000 one chief executive described how he had been phoned by Chris Ham, the head of policy in the Department of Health, and asked to provide a list of ten financial freedoms that trusts would enjoy, ready for consideration by the Secretary of State the next morning. His director of finance drew up a list on the train and the following day its contents were on the minister's desk. This back-of-an-envelope approach formed the basis for a new policy of freeing hospitals from central control and handing them back powers and freedoms that they had not enjoyed since before 1948.

A powerful group of six chief executives, analogous to the Russell Group of top university vice-chancellors, was quickly formed. Over the course of the next three years the six intensified their relationship with the health policy adviser at 10 Downing Street and with the Secretary of State personally, pressing for less control, less civil service bureaucracy and much greater freedoms. Just as in the 1940s, these representatives of the big teaching hospitals were once again in a position to put their mark on the distribution of resources and the pattern of hospital organisation. They had already had a taste of the private sector in formulating PFI schemes. Now they wanted to get rid of the remaining civil service structures that still limited their autonomy. In 2003 the Secretary of State, John Reid, responded by announcing a further dramatic downsizing of the Department of Health, reducing its establishment by 38 per cent.[83] In the new dispensation the Department's remaining capacity to plan for and secure the provision of health services to meet population needs would be less and less required. What happened in future was to be decided by the market.

As for introducing private providers into the NHS, the civil service had been increasingly focused on privatisation for more than a decade. There was even a Department of Health section responsible for capacity, plurality and the 'patient choice' programme, charged with 'growing' the private health care sector. Now the government signalled a more radical change:[84] the last vestiges of the NHS's planning structures were to go. As we saw in Chapter 3, district health authorities had already been abolished and replaced with 'strategic health authorities' (which are themselves destined for abolition once all or most hospital and other NHS trusts have aquired foundation status). Now a full hospital care market was to be created, at least for suppliers, through a further key change in the way hospitals were to be funded, opening up hospital care to private sector provision.

FROM A 'NATIONAL TARIFF' TO RISK-ADJUSTED PRICING

The 'national tariff' announced in 2003 will require all NHS hospitals to charge identical fixed prices for treatments commissioned by their purchasers (i.e. the primary care trusts). These prices are linked to an average length of stay. From the point of view of the private health care industry, however, this fixed price system involves risks they are disinclined to take. A patient needing a hip replacement might be an otherwise very healthy sixty-year-old, or he or she might be a seventy-five-year-old with diabetes. The costs of treating the two patients are liable to be widely different. An NHS district general hospital is in theory obliged to take on all patients, so that high-cost patients are balanced by low-cost patients. But a private company entering the government's new 'mixed economy of health care' market cannot rely on this happening. To make a profit and avoid a loss they want to be sure that every case they take on will be priced at roughly what it is going to cost to treat it, plus a profit. So if the government wanted for-profit providers to take over a significant part of the NHS's hospital work, the national tariff would have to change to a system of pricing according to the different 'risk categories' into which patients fell. It might make a mockery of rational medicine and integrated care, but it is the logic of pricing.

And so in 2001 the government announced that it would fund the development of a new methodology designed to allow health care providers to adjust their prices according to the risks of care.[85] In other words the state itself was working out a way to segment the population into different risk groups so that providers could set their prices according to the risks they took on. This method of risk adjustment, known as 'case mix adjustment', was pioneered in the USA. Each treatment is priced according to the risk group a patient belongs to: the healthy sixty-year-old candidate for a hip replacement will fall in one category, and the seventy-year-old with diabetes and heart disease in another. Now both purchasers and providers would be able to take steps to insure themselves against a patient costing more than the average by charging appropriately. But the government, while implementing the system across the NHS, was careful to exempt private sector providers of NHS services. Evidence to the Health Select Committee showed that private sector providers were being given 40 per cent above the average NHS cost for treating patients, having also been allowed to select only standard types of low-cost, high-turnover procedures.[86]

What is so mind-boggling about the decision to adopt risk-adjusted pricing is that it flies in the face of the findings of an enormous literature which shows that when this system is in place providers are in effect bound either to try to avoid taking on the risks, or to claim a higher price for greater risk by trying to change the categories patients are said to fall under.[87] (The Department of Health was careful to cite this evidence in the appendix of its report on risk-adjusted pricing, but it nevertheless continued to implement the policy.) In the USA, for example, 'DRG drift' is the name of a scam whereby the insurer or government is invoiced for a treatment for a patient that falls into a higher-risk, and therefore higher-price, category (Diagnosis Related Group, or DRG) than has actually been performed. For example a simple varicose veins operation is upgraded to a more complex procedure. The modern history of the US medical insurance industry and health maintenance organisations (HMOs) – including the so-called 'non-profits' – shows this practice to be virtually universal.

The private health insurance industry everywhere reduces its risk by screening out high-risk groups or by charging extra premiums – i.e. 'cherry-picking' or 'cream-skimming'. Anyone who reaches the age of sixty-five or who has a chronic illness, or predisposition to illness, for example, sees their private health insurance premiums increase dramatically, and it is common practice for private health care and private health insurance companies to exclude entirely certain predictable categories of need – for example diabetes – or to put a ceiling on the amount of care they will pay for. The Superman actor, Christopher Reeves, who became quadriplegic in a riding accident, discovered that his health care insurance had a cap on catastrophic illness, leaving him liable. Private hospitals offer a limited menu of treatments, and to a limited range of people, carefully selecting the treatments and patients they want and finding ways of excluding high-risk groups.

In the USA even non-profit HMOs are universally loathed because in order to stay afloat financially they too bend the rules, lie, 'lose' documentation and engage in a hundred other tricks to avoid taking on, or covering the actual costs of, higher-risk patients. There is no reason to think that foundation trusts, with strong incentives to maximise returns and minimise costs, and not subject to supervision by the strategic health authorities, will behave altogether differently.

A 'MIXED ECONOMY OF CARE'

By the time the Labour government had completed its first term of office it had resurrected most of the structures of a market-oriented system and the stage was set for more reform. The *NHS Plan* of 2000 outlined in Chapter 3 was premised on far greater autonomy for hospitals and much more rigorous exposure to market forces. Labour now proposed to push privatisation into the core of the NHS by bringing competing private providers into the NHS hospital sector. NHS patients will in future be treated by a diversity of providers, including domestic and overseas for-profit companies and the voluntary sector, as well as by NHS hospitals. The publicly funded NHS will still pay for health care, but independent corporations of one type or another will increasingly provide it. The role of government is to be reduced to that of payer, while the provider role is increasingly assumed by for-profit corporations.

The new roles already announced for the private sector include providing spare hospital capacity, performing up to 150,000 procedures a year; providing management to run failing NHS hospital trusts; forming joint ventures with NHS organisations; and providing clinical teams from abroad for existing NHS providers or for new NHS-managed developments. Overseas companies as well as domestic ones will be able to provide any of these services, paid for by the NHS.

The government also started contracting out NHS elective surgery to hospitals in mainland Europe. In 2002, 190 patients from three NHS sites in southern England (East Kent, Portsmouth & Isle of Wight, and West Sussex & East Surrey) were sent on pilot schemes for elective care at a hospital in Lille, France; eight more were sent to hospitals and a day-care centre in northern Germany.[88] Other patients at risk of breaching waiting-time targets for cardiac surgery or other urgent treatments may be sent to Germany, Belgium, Italy and Spain.[89]

Another entry point for private enterprise has been created by inviting private companies to manage 'failing' NHS hospital trusts. Three of the eight NHS hospitals that failed to achieve any 'stars' in the government's review of hospital performance in July 2002 were to be run by private management companies under three-year contracts. The Royal United Hospital Trust in Bath, the United Bristol Healthcare Trust in Bristol, and the Good Hope Hospital Trust in Birmingham were the first to be franchised out. Eight private sector corporations were given the right to bid: BUPA and BMI, Britain's largest hospital groups; the Swedish-owned Capio; Interhealth Canada; Hospitalia Active Health from Germany; the British-owned facilities management company Serco; Secta Group, and the consultancy firm Quo Health (both British). Few of these had previous experience of running hospitals before, and of those that had, most had never run organisations as complex as NHS hospitals, which are at least ten times the size and far more complex than a typical private hospital specialising in elective surgery.

And now for the first time since 1948 a medical career entirely outside the NHS – though funded by it – began to be potentially attractive to consultants. In 2001 the BMA published guidance for hospital doctors considering exchanging their salaried status for that of subcontractors and forming doctors' 'chambers', on the model of barristers' chambers, as a way in which to sell their services to the NHS and other hospital providers. Under this arrangement, primary care trusts could buy hospital doctors' medical services separately from the hospital infrastructure. If chambers go ahead, hospital services in Britain will have come close to full circle, reverting to something similar to the pre-1948 situation, when consultants 'visited' the voluntary hospitals run by independent charities. The difference, however, is that chambers are likely to be financed by venture capitalists and run by multinational health care companies.

FOUNDATION TRUSTS

But the most radical and controversial of all the new measures involved turning NHS hospitals into independent 'public interest corporations' with so-called 'foundation' status, described in Chapter 3. The proposals were drawn up by the UK government and its policy advisers, who included the former chief executive and aides of the Californian HMO Kaiser Permanente, and representatives of private sector pressure groups such as the Institute of Directors.[90] Foundation-status organisations will have NHS assets transferred to their ownership and control. They will be freed from NHS oversight via the strategic health authorities and be subject only to an independent regulator, who will be primarily concerned with their financial viability. Their directors will be accountable not to the Secretary of State for Health but to boards consisting of hospital managers and representatives of the hospital staff and patients and local residents. They will have the power to set their own terms and conditions of service, freedom to borrow for capital investment, freedom to generate income, and freedom to retain the proceeds of land sales.

The Secretary of State has emphasised the idea of 'community ownership' in relation to the boards. Ian McCartney, the chair of the Labour Party's National Policy Forum, called foundation hospitals 'a new form of public ownership', adding that this proposal has moved 'the debate about who should own public assets away from Thatcher's popular capitalism'. These hospitals, he said:

> ... cannot be described as 'elitist' in any real sense of the word.... They lock the public resources of the hospital into ownership by the citizen in the community: owned by the community, for the community, serving the community. ... This is public ownership, which means exactly that: owned by the public.[91]

But as critics of the Bill argued, and a close examination of its provisions shows (see p. 72), this claim was grossly misleading. If the 1962 Hospital Plan was the high point in the evolution of the NHS, the introduction of foundation trusts marks its virtual demise. Foundation trust status restores power to the vested interests of the big teaching hospitals and the acute hospital sector generally. It finally disposes of the systems that had gradually been established to secure local accountability, needs-based planning and fairness in resource allocation. Nominally responding to market signals and delivering business-style efficiencies, foundation trusts will in reality constitute a state-funded hierarchy of political power, led by the teaching hospital elite and their increasingly powerful and vocal friends in the for-profit and voluntary sectors. In an interview in July 2000 the chief spokesperson of the Independent Healthcare Association foresaw a time when the NHS would be simply a 'kitemark', attached to the institutions and activities of a system of purely private providers.[92] He could hardly have imagined how quickly this vision would start to become a reality.

5

PRIMARY CARE

Most of the media attention given to the NHS focuses on the daily drama of hospitals, the high-tech advances in medicine and surgery, and busy Accident and Emergency departments. But most people's everyday experience of the NHS is at their GP's surgery, and it can be argued that the provision of 24-hour general medical services for the entire population was the NHS's single greatest achievement. Whereas before 1948 you could get basic medical attention only if you were an insured working man, or had enough income to pay a doctor's fee, under the NHS every family became entitled to basic medical attention as of right.

Yet unlike hospital doctors, GPs remained technically outside the NHS, choosing to be 'independent contractors' to the government, rather than salaried. This made it difficult for the architects of the NHS to achieve the integration between health promotion and curing illnesses, and between GPs' services and hospital services, that they understood to be crucial to good population health. Their hope had been that GPs would lead primary care teams (including other health care professionals such as practice nurses, physiotherapists, chiropodists, dieticians and counsellors, as well as support staff) in purpose-built, publicly owned health centres. Instead most GPs continued to work alone, mostly in more or less inadequate premises owned by themselves. Other NHS primary care services gradually grew up alongside them, but proper integration remained elusive.

Today the single-handed GP is becoming rare – over 90 per cent now work in group practices with two or more other doctors – and their premises are better. Some surgeries are still in Victorian houses or Georgian tenements, often in dire need of modernisation, but more are in Portacabin-like functional buildings of more recent construction, and some are in architect-designed premises very like the health centres envisaged by the pre-1948 proponents of integrated primary care. More and more of the larger practice premises now also accommodate a variety of other primary care practitioners, from pharmacists to physiotherapists and district nurses. They also often house specialist primary care services, including clinics for the management of chronic diseases such as diabetes, asthma and heart disease (services increasingly transferred to primary care from hospitals), and facilities for preventive work such as child health clinics, immunisations and cervical screening. Changes in clinical practice, including shorter lengths of stay in hospital, the closure of long-stay NHS institutions, and new drugs and treatments mean that GPs now offer a wider range of care to a larger population pool than ever before. And some GPs have begun to accept salaried employment after all.

But ironically, just as the vision of integrated primary care might seem capable of being achieved, GPs are surrendering their dominant role in primary care. Control over the direction of primary care now belongs to PCTs, and increasingly the corporate sector. Although GPs were supposed to play the leading role in the PCTs, in practice this has not happened. GPs are also giving up more and more elements of the comprehensive family care they used to provide, which is being taken over by a diverse range of other providers, from 'walk-in clinics' to specialist on-call services, with a resulting loss of continuity of care. Corporate owners of general practice premises, and some corporate primary care providers, are playing an increasing role in shaping the evolution of primary care. As a result, even though PCTs nominally control 75 per cent of the NHS budget (see page 51), it is not clear that they will be able to secure the integration of primary care with hospital and other services that this control might lead one to expect. Instead, what is emerging is a pattern of primary care based on market principles, in which priorities will be increasingly set by criteria of profitability, not the equal provision of comprehensive health care to all who need it.

It might be thought that this was a predictable outcome of the GPs' 'independent contractor' status, but in reality GPs embraced the NHS's founding values more and more fully over the years. How primary care has finally been pushed in an overtly commercial direction can only be understood by looking briefly at how general practice was painfully detached from its unrewarding origins as a market activity half a century ago.

THE ORIGINS OF GENERAL PRACTICE

In Victorian Britain, workers clubbed together to contract with an individual GP to provide them with basic medical services for a monthly fee. This guaranteed GPs an income, but it was not a good income, and the 'sick club' system only covered working men: women and children and the unemployed were not provided for. In 1911 National Insurance, funded by contributions from employers and the state as well as workers, largely replaced voluntary insurance. It was compulsory for workers earning less than £160 a year, and its benefits extended to include cash payments for workers when they were sick or unemployed. But 21 million people, mainly the wives and children of working men, were still not covered.[1]

Under National Insurance the fee per enrolled patient, or 'capitation fee' paid by the state to GPs, was double the payment they had received from the voluntary societies, and the number of patients on their lists greatly expanded too, which undoubtedly led to improvements in GP services as well as GPs' incomes.[2] On the other hand the new system allowed GPs to remain self-employed practitioners, maintaining the right to own and sell their practices, and to take on private patients. And while the ability to diagnose illnesses steadily advanced, until the advent of antibiotics in the 1940s the range of available treatments remained limited. A famous NHS GP, Julian Tudor Hart, later summed up the change rather wryly: 'the doctor, unconvincingly disguised as a scientific gentleman, remained a shopkeeper; but a shopkeeper paid increasingly by the state rather than customers'.[3]

Besides not covering women and children, the National Insurance scheme also did not cover hospital care. But in 1944, with the war on the way to being won, the wartime government announced that it would underwrite the costs of a universal health care system, covering the whole population and all medical care, and funded entirely by central taxation.

Earlier thinking about such a system had envisaged a unified and comprehensive health service in which curative and preventive medicine would be integrated, and had included the idea of 'health centres'. As early as 1920 the Consultative Council on Medical and Allied Services, chaired by Lord Dawson of Penn, produced an interim report that advocated the establishment of health centres, arguing that

> preventive and curative medicine cannot be separated on any sound principle, and in any scheme of medical services must be brought together in close co-ordination. They must likewise be brought within the sphere of the general practitioner, whose duties should embrace the work of communal as well as industrial medicine.[4]

Dawson envisaged that local authorities would be responsible for primary health care centres – in effect general practitioner centres that would also provide a range of other services including dental, pharmaceutical and ophthalmic care. Each centre would be staffed by six to twelve doctors. The state would pay GPs a basic salary plus a capitation fee related to the number of patients on their lists, and additional payments for special qualifications and length of service, plus fees for services that fell outside the usual terms.

The health centre idea was put into practice in the Peckham Health Centre in 1935 and the Finsbury Health Centre in 1938,[5] and Dawson's recommendations were also incorporated into the 1944 White Paper *A National Health Service*.[6] This proposed the creation of a Central Medical Board which would employ GPs and also be able to prohibit new doctors from practising in areas where there were already too many. Apart from the proposal of a Central Medical Board, which was dropped, with some modifications all these ideas were included in the National Health Service Bill of March 1946, which additionally proposed that the sale and purchase of GP practices should be prohibited.

Younger GPs were in favour of these proposals: a BMA poll conducted in 1944 found that 83 per cent of GPs in the armed services were in favour of a salaried service and health centres,[7] and another survey in 1948 found that 89 per cent of medical students agreed.[8] But the BMA leadership, speaking for older and established GPs, were vehemently opposed to the introduction of even a basic salary.[9] They wanted to continue to be paid by capitation and believed a basic salary would threaten traditional professional freedoms and limit their ability to undertake private practice. They also wanted to go on being able to buy and sell their practices, and feared having their income entirely dependent on government, be it local or national. An accommodation was eventually reached. GPs continued to be paid by capitation and remained independent. But the costs to the profession of not becoming a salaried service were high. In stark contrast to their salaried hospital colleagues, GPs, because of their independent status, continued to carry significant financial risks. As well as the normal risks of owning the practice premises, GPs had to cover the costs arising from the need to employ locums to cover any periods when they themselves were sick (maternity and paternity leave and illness can have a severely adverse impact on a practice, even though GPs insure against it; they enjoy none of the protections afforded to direct employees of the state). Although GPs continued to own their own premises, the NHS Act did outlaw the sale and purchase of the 'goodwill' attached to practices – the element in the sale price of a business that reflects the income it has generated and is expected to generate in the future. In other words the idea that patients had a commercial value was abolished. The government set aside £66 million as compensation, but to receive it the 17,700 established GPs had to sign a contract with the NHS.

So although the NHS was established with the aim of integrating cure with prevention, hospital care with primary care, and general practice with public health, political realities blocked the achievement of this ideal. Yet the battle for integration and a salaried GP service was not over.

INEQUALITIES IN PRIMARY CARE AND THE CONTINUED DEBATE OVER HEALTH CENTRES

When the NHS came into existence in July 1948, the geographical distribution of primary care resources was highly inequitable: as the

American observer Harry Eckstein put it, 'places such as Harrogate were gorged with doctors while working class areas nearby in cities such as Wakefield, Leeds and Bradford were comparatively starved. Kensington had seven times as many doctors per unit of population as South Shields'.[10] Four years later, in 1952, GP list sizes in the North of England, the East and the West Midlands still averaged 2,700 compared with just over 2,200 in the Southwest and Scotland.[11] To remedy this the government did finally establish a Medical Practices Committee (MPC), which defined areas as 'over-doctored', 'intermediate' or 'under-doctored', and barred new entrants from practising in over-doctored areas. This proved effective. In just seven years, from 1951 to 1958, the proportion of the population of England and Wales living in 'under-doctored' areas fell from 51 per cent to 19 per cent.[12] But the basic problem of integrating general practice with other elements of health care remained.

Moreover, a survey of fifty-five English practices outside London found that their standards varied widely and unacceptably.[13] Practices often lacked such basic facilities as an examination couch. Some surgeries were even in condemned buildings, and the worst were located where the need was greatest, in areas of deprivation and dense population. GPs had no source of revenue other than their own incomes with which to invest in improvements, and therefore little incentive to do so.

In 1950 the Ministry of Health commissioned a wide-ranging review of the role of general practice within the NHS.[14] Chaired by Sir Henry Cohen, a professor of medicine in Liverpool, the review committee recommended independent GP group practices as a superior alternative to local-authority-owned health centres on the grounds that group practices would be better able to secure premises, staff and equipment. Local authority health centres were said to be unpopular with GPs because the rents were high and they took too long to design and build. The Treasury's reluctance to make capital funds available was a further factor militating against publicly owned health centres.

The turning-point in the health centre debate finally came with the 1952 GPs' pay settlement adjudicated by Harold Danckwerts, a High Court Judge, which attempted to deal with GPs' status, pay and practice premises together.[15] To remedy the widely held view that hospital specialists had higher status than GPs, Danckwerts proposed reducing the pay gap between them, and also recommended the provision of interest-free loans for GPs to help them develop their practice premises. The Treasury, alarmed by rising NHS expenditure, much preferred a loans scheme to a large programme of capital grants for health centres, and as a result the solution to the poor quality of GP premises came to be seen as group practices rather than health centres.

The Danckwerts settlement also gave a financial incentive for the formation of group practices, and this, together with the new loans for GP premises, stimulated their expansion.[16] In 1952 there were 7,459 single-handed GPs, while 9,745 practised in partnerships. By 1956, 12,272 GPs were in partnerships, an increase of 30 per cent, while the number of single-handers had fallen by 10 per cent.[17]

GROUP PRACTICES AND THE 1966 FAMILY DOCTORS CHARTER

By 1964 the correspondence columns of medical journals were full of letters from GPs complaining about their terms of service. For the first time the number of GPs fell, and it continued to fall for the next two years. In 1965 nearly 18,000 GPs – about 75 per cent of the total – who were unhappy with their remuneration threatened mass resignation. The BMA called for a 'charter' for the family doctor service: an entirely new contract that would not only allow GPs a choice of methods to finance and pay for practice premises, but also reduce the maximum list size to 2,000 patients and limit the GP's working day. The eventual result was the Family Doctors Charter, adopted by the government and the BMA in 1966. The capitation or flat fee would be higher for patients over sixty-five; a basic practice allowance would be paid, which would be greater for group practices and practices in unattractive areas; and payments would also be made for GPs' seniority. The charter was a political endorsement of the group practice model, and finally set the seal on the model of GPs as independent contractors and owner-occupiers.

A crucially important element of the Family Doctors Charter was that the Treasury created an Independent Finance Corporation (subsequently called the General Practice Finance Corporation or GPFC) from which GPs could borrow money to buy land, construct new premises, or convert existing ones. In effect GPs were subsidised, as the GPFC lent money at a lower rate than private lenders. The Family Doctors Charter also established the principle of reimbursing GPs for the cost of servicing their capital debt – i.e. the public now paid for GPs' premises, even though GPs continued to own them. The new loan scheme enabled a huge expansion of purpose-built or adapted premises, and encouraged group practice by allowing GPs to share services in them. The high cost that had previously been a barrier to building premises was now no longer a charge against GPs' personal incomes. In fact GPs in some areas did very well out of the schemes. Reimbursement was also provided for 70 per cent of the expenses of practice staff, which led to the employment of additional staff such as receptionists and nurses.

All these changes raised the quality of primary care and accelerated the trend towards group practice, and the numbers of doctors taking up general practice rose again. Yet it was also at this time that significant amounts of public capital finally became available for constructing local authority health centres. From 1967 to 1977 no less than 700 publicly owned health centres were built, compared with only 28 in the nineteen years from 1948 to 1967.[18] At this point, the integration of GP and other services in health centres still seemed to be a path that primary care might conceivably take.

But the subsequently adopted policy of 'care in the community', and the closure of large institutions, although positive in its intentions, was not accompanied by sufficient extra resources. Inevitably the extra work fell on GPs. Looking at new ways to cope with the demand for their services by running their practices differently, GPs introduced appointment systems and spent less time visiting patients at home, encouraging them to come to the surgery instead – a trend that continues to this day. But home visits are a very important part of family medicine because they are an important means by which GPs can gain insight into the living conditions and family arrangements, and therefore the service needs, of their patients. Nevertheless, GPs were increasingly conscious of their need for continuing post-qualification training. The Royal College of General Practitioners, formed in 1952, introduced specialist vocational training for GPs, and in 1984 this became mandatory and began to make the education, training and standards of care offered by GPs comparable to those of hospital specialists. The profession was taking account of criticisms both from within and from without.

A 'PRIMARY-CARE-LED' NHS AND THE SHIFT TO A 'MIXED ECONOMY' OF CARE

Although in some areas a degree of integration of GP services with local authority health services had occurred during the 1950s and 1960s through the formation of 'primary care teams', progress was limited; and virtually no integration had been achieved between primary care and the hospital sector, making it difficult to accommodate the new demands for health services that were constantly emerging. For example the rising burden of chronic diseases such as diabetes and heart disease, and the trend to treating more and more patients 'in the community', required a much greater degree of co-ordination of care, and more information-sharing, between hospital specialists and GPs. GPs were still often considered inferior to their hospital consultant counterparts and communication was (and continues to be) a perennial problem. Similarly the organisational and funding division between primary care and community-based nursing, public health, and social services posed major difficulties for the delivery of integrated care. Successive reorganisations of the administrative structure of the NHS were attempted during the 1970s with a view to overcoming some of these structural problems, but so long as GPs remained outside the jurisdiction of the district health authorities, reorganisations achieved little.

Nevertheless, during the 1980s primary care increasingly became the focus of attention because policy-makers anxious to control NHS public spending, 60 per cent of which was on hospital and community health services, began to realise that GPs could be the key to implementing cost containment policies.[19] This was for two reasons. First, GPs were the gatekeepers to hospital care, since apart from referrals via Accident and Emergency departments a hospital specialist could only see patients referred by a GP. Second, whereas the hospitals budget was directly controlled by the Department of Health, the money GPs spent was not, and the amount was escalating – especially the cost of prescription drugs, which accounted for nearly half of the total cost of family medical services. So successive governments began to argue that patients – meaning, in practice, their GPs – should be 'at the heart' of decision-making in the NHS, while at the same time the need for accountability in primary care was increasingly emphasised. And although there was no way of imposing cash limits on GPs' expenditure without renegotiating the GP contract, in 1984 the Conservative government did limit the list of drugs for which it would reimburse GPs, in spite of the conflict this was bound to generate.

So in the 1990s GPs increasingly found themselves promoted to the driving seat – or so it appeared – of NHS reform. At the same time there continued to be significant shifts in workload from hospitals to GPs, without an adequate transfer of resources. In particular the management of maternity services and chronic diseases such as diabetes, and heart and lung disease, which had traditionally been the responsibility of hospital-based specialists, now rested with GPs, but without the nursing and administrative support that hospital doctors had enjoyed for this work.

GP fundholding

One of the most acrimonious public battles fought within the NHS was over GP fundholding. As we saw in Chapter 3, the NHS and Community Care Act of 1990 made district health authorities into 'purchasers' of care from hospitals and community services (the 'providers'), creating the so-called purchaser/provider split, or internal market. But it also introduced GP fundholding, under which GPs in larger practices were allocated budgets to 'purchase' hospital treatment or community care, such as outpatient services, diagnostic tests, and some non-emergency inpatient services, for the patients on their lists.

Fundholding divided GPs. Originally, there was little support for fundholding except from the most Thatcherite of GPs. GPs had by now become part and parcel of the NHS – they valued the principles and philosophy that for all the NHS's faults allowed them to practise excellent family medicine. As independent practitioners they understood only too well what the reintroduction of market principles would do to health care. The BMA mobilised and launched an extraordinary public campaign to oppose Kenneth Clarke, the Secretary of State for Health. GPs lost no time in informing their patients; and many practices, especially in the East End of London, sent huge petitions to Downing Street. But the government pressed ahead, disregarding the BMA's well-articulated objections and using a few GP supporters as product champions. The BMA was defeated, leaving its membership divided. The BMA would never again challenge the government on a matter of principle.

By 1991 the new market mechanisms were already producing the effects critics had predicted. GP fundholders and non-fundholders had organised themselves into two distinct camps and with two different organisations to support them. Early fundholders, especially, enjoyed the power *vis-à-vis* hospital consultants that the ability to negotiate their own contracts for hospital services gave them, and some were inclined to dismiss their non-fundholding colleagues' concerns over the loss of equity between patients.

GP fundholding was a voluntary scheme, and to get it adopted the Conservative government introduced financial incentives that allowed fundholding GPs to keep any surpluses they accumulated and invest them in their premises or use them to purchase new equipment, or take on new staff. Fundholders could also finance new services such as counselling and physiotherapy and consultant outreach clinics, as they were able to transfer any budgetary savings between the different components of patient care as they wished. For GPs, fundholding represented extra funding and greater access to hospital-based investigations (such as exercise tests for diagnosing heart disease, x-rays and imaging for a range of conditions from bone fractures to suspected cancer, and endoscopies for detecting gastro-intestinal disorders), and it also tended to reduce waiting times for hospital outpatient appointments for their patients. Fundholding GPs were free to choose the type of hospital care their patients should receive, and where. Increasingly fundholding GPs would also buy services from the private sector.

The payments made under fundholding differed significantly from those that GPs had previously received. Under the capitation system – a flat rate for every patient on a GP's list and allowances linked to staff and premises costs – GPs only had to cover the costs of running the practice, including salary costs for nurses and other practice staff. No other costs of providing care, including the costs of prescription drugs, fell on GPs. But under fundholding, GPs had a budget to manage, including a budget for the cost of prescriptions and a budget for purchasing care, such as elective surgery in hospital. Consequently, in theory at least, if the costs of patient care in a given year exceeded the budget, the financial cost was borne by the practice, which could lead to decisions affecting patients having to be made on financial instead of clinical grounds.

These risks were heightened by the fact that fundholding meant abandoning, up to a point, one of the NHS's great advantages: the wide pooling of risk. Within the NHS the risks of falling ill and needing treatment, and so incurring costs, had been shared, in principle, across the entire UK – for very rare conditions – or at least across the whole population covered by one of the 100 district health authorities. Under fundholding, the risk was only spread over the patients registered in a single practice, i.e. some 11,000 patients, or even less as fundholding was extended to smaller and smaller practices. The risks were increased, too, as the scope of fundholding was expanded to cover all elective surgery, hospital outpatient care, psychiatric care, and specialist nursing services. A limit was placed on these risks: if any patient of a fundholding practice incurred costs of more than £5,000, the district health authority covered the extra cost. Such patients, however, were the exception. For all the others fundholding GPs had to manage their budgets so that they did not end the year with a deficit, which could encourage GPs to under-treat some patients in favour of others, or decline to accept new patients whom they judged likely to be relatively high users of primary care, such as the very old.

But the most important risk that fundholders accepted was the cost of prescriptions. Hitherto GPs' independent status meant that they could prescribe freely, and the district health authority would pick up the bill.[20] Under fundholding, however, the full cost of prescriptions was included in the fundholding budget and the GPs involved had to police each others' prescribing or end up in debt.

The government was then left with the non-fundholding practices, whose prescription bills continued to rise. To bring them into line with fundholding practices the government set 'indicative prescribing' budgets, based mainly on a practice's past pattern of expenditure. GPs were able to keep half of any savings on their prescribing bill, to spend on equipment or improving their premises. Although GPs feared this would put financial considerations before clinical need, the principle of setting cash-limited budgets for general practice had come to stay.[21]

By the late 1990s over half of all GPs in Britain were fundholders, and fundholding practices accounted for 15 per cent of all hospital and community health service income. Nevertheless there was deep public and political hostility to fundholding. The small risk pools and the high 'transaction costs' involved in the negotiation of hundreds of contracts between fundholders and providers made the system ultimately unviable, and the two-tier system of family medicine it was creating was too visible. The early financial benefits from fundholding were also available only to larger group practices, which were already better resourced and better able to take advantage of the early windfalls than the rest. Empirical evidence on the consequences of fundholding is sparse, but anecdotal accounts repeatedly suggested that fundholding gave fundholders' patients better access to hospital care than patients of non-fundholding GPs, because fundholders were able to make fast and better access a condition for awarding a purchasing contract to a hospital.[22] The evidence also suggests that non-fundholders received fewer resources than fundholders for both inpatient and outpatient care.[23]

The early or 'first wave' fundholders enjoyed their new-found leverage over their hospital consultant colleagues and the hospitals themselves. For the first time in the history of the NHS, GPs were in the driving seat, with the power to move resources and income around to meet their patients' needs. The problem was, however, that GPs lacked both the skills and the incentive to take a population-oriented perspective and to safeguard planning and access for all. Those skills and that outlook were located in the district health authorities, but as these authorities came to be seen as merely purchasers of services, rather than as providers and planners, their expert staff were made redundant.

Primary care trusts

When Labour came to power in 1997 it announced the abolition of fundholding, to almost universal approval, although a position as National Clinical Director for Primary Care in England was given to Dr David Colin-Thome, a prominent GP fundholder. And the primary care trusts introduced by Labour in 2002 actually consolidated the idea of the market principles underlying fundholding, extending it to all GPs and all hospital and community services. Each PCT included all the practices in an area covering, by 2003, an average population of 170,000; through their role in the PCT GPs were now supposed to become the key NHS decision-makers, exercising many of the responsibilities that had formerly belonged to the district health authority. Together the PCTs became theoretically responsible for spending 75 per cent of the total NHS budget, including buying all hospital services for the patients in their areas.[24]

In reality, however, the new PCT structures diluted rather than strengthened the power of GPs, as the full pattern of New Labour's market-oriented reforms began to take shape. GPs, having helped in paving the way for market-oriented reforms, would now be relegated to the back seat again. The government had no interest in small corner-shop entrepreneurs – its interest was now in developing the health care industry as an international competitor. The question was how best to do this. Eventually, corporate capital was brought in through a new kind of PFI scheme for practice premises, LIFT, described below. However there was as yet no mechanism for making primary care services them-selves into a field of interest to corporate capital – if anything, GPs' role in primary care had expanded, and their control over staff and services had been consolidated during the fundholding era. Before this could be changed the GPs' General Medical Services (GMS) contract had to be renegotiated yet again.

The beginning of the end of GPs' monopoly of primary care

This renegotiation was facilitated by the fact that the NHS (Primary Care) Act of 1997 had in the meantime introduced a new kind of optional GP contract, called Personal Medical Services (PMS).[25] Under a PMS contract individual GPs, or whole practices, or groups of prac-tices, could negotiate terms and conditions of service locally with their district health authority, though following national rules, with payment based on meeting set quality standards and accounting for population needs. The aim of PMS was to improve GP recruitment, particularly in deprived areas, by offering GPs more flexible forms of employment.

It had become increasingly hard to recruit new GPs in urban areas, especially to replace those who were due to retire, or who were seeking early retirement; and in 2000 one in three GPs was over fifty.[26] With a PMS contract, GPs could maintain their personal patient lists and keep their independent contractor status; but they also had the option of becoming salaried employees – the very thing GP leaders had fought so hard against in 1946. By 2000 some 28 per cent of GPs had switched to PMS, and over half the pilot PMS schemes were for salaried employment.[27]

A study of forty-six 'first-wave' PMS pilot schemes showed, however, that salaried employment was not a magic solution to all the recruitment and retention problems facing general practice.[28] Moreover local contracts opened up the possibility of a widening of regional disparities in GP pay and in the level and type of primary care that GPs provided, and did little to address the problem of unequal access to GPs across the UK.

But a key feature of the PMS contract was that whether or not GPs chose to be salaried they were no longer reimbursed for the costs they actually incurred in providing care. Now they received a practice budget, usually paid on a monthly basis, in return for achieving specified results. As in fundholding, GPs with PMS contracts became responsible for managing the financial risks of delivering care.

The PMS contract option also opened up the possibility of using new mixes of skills in primary care, expanding the roles and responsibilities of other professional groups including nurses, managers and therapists, and ending the traditional demarcation of roles and responsibilities in service provision. The government was keen to address the continuing problem of recruiting and retaining GPs by transferring some of their workload to nurses and other health professionals. Following the changes in the last GP contract in 1990, nurses had already begun to undertake more aspects of primary care, such as treating patients with minor illnesses and running health promotion and asthma clinics; now, under some PMS contracts, nurses even employed GPs. Pharmacists were now also increasingly employed by PCTs to help manage prescribing budgets and to deliver some components of care.

The new GP contract of 2002

It was in the context of these broader changes that a new GP contract was negotiated. A crucial element of the first GP contract established in 1948 had been the provision by GPs of 24-hour, 365-days-a-year medical cover for all registered patients. But GPs can now arrange far more services for patients than was possible in 1948, and they have also become responsible for new elements of care, such as undertaking health promotion, minor surgery and managing patients with chronic diseases, mental illness or diseases of addiction, that were formerly provided in hospitals. The rising workload this involved made GPs increasingly ready to reduce their contractual obligations to a core set of services. In particular, many were happy to give up their commitment to provide care 24 hours a day, which had been a key characteristic of UK family medicine. This reflected the fact that by the mid 1990s GPs' working patterns had begun to alter dramatically. The rise in patient workload and the reluctance of more and more GPs to provide 24-hour care had already led them to reorganise the provision of 'out-of-hours' cover, mainly through expanding GP co-operatives and by contracting with commercial 'deputising' services to provide it. The trend towards larger partnerships had also intensified: in the decade from 1990 to 2000 the number of single-handed GPs in England continued to fall, from 2,975 to 2,575 – i.e. to only 9.3 per cent of the total.[29]

These changes in turn reflected the fact that there were now many more women GPs – by 2000 one in three GP principals (i.e. those providing general medical services, as opposed to, say, working for a company) was a woman – and that one in five GPs worked part-time. Especially among younger GPs, who were predominantly women, there was a desire for salaried employment and flexible working hours.

The new UK GP contract of April 2002 was the biggest shake-up of NHS primary care since 1948.[30] It signified the end of general practitioners' monopoly over the provision of primary care services, transferring the control of and accountability for primary care services from GPs to primary care trusts and signalling the increasing dominance of market forces over the pattern of service delivery.

From April 2004 onwards, contracts would be negotiated between PCTs and general practices, not between the Secretary of State and individual GPs through the BMA. National terms and conditions of service were also abolished, paving the way for local pay bargaining and widening inequities in pay. As part of this process GPs' personal lists were also abolished; patients are now registered with the practice in which their GPs work. GPs were also made accountable to their practices and to PCTs by a series of market-based financial incentives linking remuneration to performance and quality.

The 1990 contract had already set the trend in this direction, introducing target payments for cervical screening and childhood immunisations. Instead of being paid for each immunisation or cervical smear, GPs now received a payment for reaching predefined target levels, so that the risk of not achieving, for example, the immunisation of 90 per cent of the population, or the cervical screening of 80 per cent of the target category, rested with them, not the Department of Health; if they failed to reach their targets, the practice − and so in turn the GPs − lost financially. In deprived urban areas where the primary care infrastructure was poor and the population not as compliant, middle-class and health-aware as in more affluent areas, many GPs struggled to achieve even the lower target of immunising 70 per cent of children in order to earn the extra payment that came with reaching that figure. And GPs' traditional clinical freedoms were further curtailed by the inclusion of more contractual details of clinical activity than before, such as a requirement to make annual at-home checks on the health of the elderly.

Another fundamental change was in the range and level of services general practices could opt to provide and the methods for reimbursing services and remunerating GPs. As mentioned above, under the new contract practices no longer have to provide 24-hour comprehensive general medical services. The contract only guarantees that all GPs will provide a 'minimum package of healthcare', PCTs being responsible for ensuring that the rest is if necessary provided by other means. The contract defines three levels of clinical care. The first level is classed as 'essential', and must be provided by all practices. It includes those services whose provision is initiated by patients who are ill, or believe themselves to be ill, and services for patients who require terminal care. GPs will be paid a global sum for providing these essential services, plus what are now termed 'additional services', including contraceptive services, maternity services and and cervical screening (hitherto seen as key elements of general practice). GPs may, however, choose to opt out of providing such 'additional services', in which case a fixed sum is deducted from their global payment for each service not provided. This money is then available to be competed for by other providers. A third level of care, not included in practice budgets, is classed as 'enhanced' services: these include care for pregnant women during labour, and anticoagulation monitoring for certain people at risk of a stroke, and will be commissioned locally, according to a national tariff.

PCTs must ensure that all these optional services – both 'additional' and 'enhanced' – are provided in one way or another. They are free to employ salaried staff to provide the services themselves, if they can show that they can offer the same value for money as anyone else, or better; alternatively, they can commission services from various other providers. The potential to subcontract primary care services to numerous providers, however, clearly puts an end to the much-admired traditional model of UK family medicine, removing its holistic nature and giving up continuity of care. The level and type of primary care services available under the new system, and the methods of provision, seem bound to vary from place to place.

Providing 'out of hours' service also became an 'additional service'. General practices had the first refusal of providing it; if a practice chose not to do so, the PCT became responsible for finding another provider, making a deduction from the budget of the practice concerned. The private deputising service Healthcall immediately saw this as a business opportunity and proposed to establish new GP call centres in Birmingham and Sheffield.[31]

To enable PCTs to use services and staff outside the NHS the government abolished the Medical Practices Committee mechanism for securing a fair distribution of GPs and of primary care services, arguing that it could be a barrier to the entry of other providers into the market for services. The committee had been effective in reducing the proportion of the population living in 'under-doctored' areas, but the resulting distribution still did not reflect the fact that the need for GPs was much higher in some areas than others because of widely varying levels of welfare and health status.[32] Now PCTs became responsible for ensuring an equitable distribution of GPs within their own areas, and a new formula was adopted for allocating primary care resources according to the practice populations served, as opposed to the total population living in the area covered by the PCT. Although this appears equitable there are some problematic implications. First, money is allocated on the basis of registered patients only, which ignores groups who tend not to be registered, such as the homeless, travellers or refugees, who tend to have more complex needs. Second, since money is to follow the patient and will no longer be linked to the number of GPs in a practice, if a GP leaves a practice the practice could try to save money by employing fewer qualified staff. The removal of national planning mechanisms and the abandonment of national norms for the services provided gives PCTs enormous latitude to determine the range, level, quality and staffing of services. Whether this market-driven conception will lead to primary care resources matching real health needs remains to be seen.

In sum, under the new contract of 2002 GPs ceased to be the dominant actors in primary care. Control was transferred to PCTs, which became agents of central government policy in a closely determined way. For example, PCTs are now responsible for supervising the 'quality' element in GPs' work. Under the new GMS contract up to one-third of GPs' incomes will come from payments for meeting performance targets in managing chronic diseases such as lung or heart disease – if they don't meet them this will have serious consequences for their incomes.

Moreover, instead of receiving funding for direct staff and premises costs, GPs now receive a 'global' budget linked to the population served by a practice. Under this system the GPs in each of the country's 11,000 practices will be responsible for providing primary care and services from a limited budget in which more than one-third of the practice income is linked to performance measures. The risks and costs of care are being passed to primary care practices without a big enough risk pool, while the introduction of draconian performance measures will see GPs trying to manage their practice lists and their services to comply with these measures rather than to meet patients' needs. At the same time if they opt out of the provision of additional or 'enhanced' services it will be in the knowledge that a range of alternative providers will be competing to provide them, driving down quality if necessary to win the business and ending the continuity of care that has been the foundation of good family practice.

NEW MARKET SUPPLIERS OF PRIMARY CARE

The new funding arrangements thus endorse the repackaging of primary care. The opening-up of primary care to new suppliers under the rubric of 'patient choice' and 'diversity' is a key element of the Labour government's policy.[33] GPs who, under the contract, opt out of providing any element of service provision will now have to compete with corporate providers if they want to opt back in. The competition includes both public and private providers.

NHS Direct and NHS walk-in centres

Both as a means of reducing the demand for GPs, and to break up the GPs' monopoly of primary care, the government introduced a new kind of gatekeeper to NHS care: NHS Direct. In effect, an important element of primary care was being reassigned to a new category of suppliers – nurses. NHS Direct is a 24-hour nurse-led telephone helpline service, established in 1998 at a cost of £80 million.[34] It claimed to provide 'easier and faster advice and information for people about health, illness and the NHS so that they are better able to care for themselves and their families'. By the end of 2000 it covered the whole of England and Wales. Scotland had its own version, called NHS 24, launched in May 2002 and initially serving the Grampian region. So far Northern Ireland has no such scheme.

NHS Direct was to be a new entry-point for 'out of hours' primary care. Directly funded and controlled by the Department of Health, it broke with the traditional GP gatekeeper model, moving to the model developed by Health Maintenance Organisations (HMOs) in the USA. There it involves 'triage' (case-prioritising) phone lines, manned by nurses who use 'decision-support' computer software to help decide whether or not to authorise patients to seek medical care, which the HMO will then pay for.[35] The question there is whether such phone lines are designed to reduce patients' access to medical services or to deliver good patient care. Patients in the USA have little doubt that it is the former. Which purpose NHS Direct will ultimately come to serve will depend on developments in the market-oriented evolution of the NHS.

NHS walk-in centres, first established in 2000, were another centrally funded government initiative run by nurses, to provide advice and information and treat patients with minor illnesses. In a way they too are a new kind of gatekeeper, since they can refer patients whose illnesses seem more serious to GPs or hospitals. By 2003, forty-two centres were open, with a further twelve due to open soon or under development. Whereas GPs are normally restricted to seeing only registered patients, so as to maintain continuity of care, walk-in centres offer you the convenience of seeing a nurse without having to make an appointment – but without the nurse knowing your medical history, or having a doctor on hand to refer you to if needed.

GPs saw both NHS Direct and NHS walk-in centres as diverting scarce resources away from themselves, and competing wastefully for the small pool of highly qualified nurses, especially in inner-city areas. It is not clear that NHS Direct or NHS walk-in centres have reduced the workload of other health care providers, such as Accident and Emergency departments or GP 'out of hours' services – the evidence is inconclusive.[36] Furthermore not all social groups use NHS Direct equally. It has tended to be chiefly used by white people under 65, and by the more socially advantaged.[37] But the chief criticism of both NHS Direct and NHS walk-in centres is that they have not been integrated with the other services they are supposed to relieve; their planning has not been based on evidence of need, and their high cost relative to efficiency has been questioned; the number of patients seen by walk-in centre staff has been relatively small, and evaluations have shown they are much more expensive than GPs' out of hours services. GPs feel that a better solution would have been to spend the major new resources devoted to this initiative directly on primary care.

OPENING UP PRIMARY CARE PROVISION TO PRIVATE SECTOR CORPORATIONS

The comprehensiveness of the old GP contract acted as an effective barrier to the private provision of primary care. After 1948 GPs had a monopoly of primary care services, but in exchange were barred from charging fees to patients on their NHS lists. If they wished, GPs could choose to practise privately, setting their own fees for seeing patients based on the market rate, but private patients had to incur the full cost of their drugs bill, which could be substantial, as GPs were not allowed to issue NHS prescriptions to these private patients. Many NHS GPs received some private income for undertaking work not covered by the GP contract, such as medical exams for insurance purposes; but in 1999–2000 only some 200 GPs were thought to be engaged in exclusively private practice and only 3 per cent of all GP consultations were estimated to be private consultations.[38] As a result private sector corporations looked at primary care as an interesting but immature market, the development of which presented a major challenge.

Private primary care insurance initiatives

An early initiative was BUPA's decision to launch a telephone-based primary care scheme in Reading in 1995, despite the restrictions imposed by NHS legislation at that time. Although this service was withdrawn three years later, other initiatives followed, responding in part to the difficulty people were experiencing at that time in getting an appointment with a GP, whether for an acute viral illness or contraceptive services. Furthermore surgery hours, which tended to be between 9am and 5pm, were inconvenient; most working people (especially younger people in city areas) wanted to see their GPs before or after work. In May 1998 Norwich Union launched the first insurance 'product' dedicated to primary health care in the UK. It offered cover for a limited number of consultations in walk-in centres, minor surgical procedures, child vaccinations and health screening, and the use of a GP helpline. The scheme was aimed at working people with families who wanted ready access to consultations for minor ailments.

An alternative scheme launched by PPP Healthcare in 2000 consisted of nominated NHS GPs who provided private primary care services to insured PPP members in return for a per capita payment; members' monthly payments varied according to age, gender and morbidity. The participating practice assumed the financial risk of both investing in new or upgraded practice facilities and providing health care to the insured patients, as in the Victorian 'sick club' system. The GPs involved meanwhile received two levels of payment for providing care – one for their private patients from PPP and one for their NHS patients from the state, creating a two-tier system within the practice. The attraction for PPP was to break into the market by employing GPs who were reluctant to leave the NHS and the guaranteed income it provided, but who welcomed the additional payments the scheme offered. For patients the attraction of the scheme was to be able to be seen by a doctor more quickly.

Primary care in retail chains

Supermarkets too have been looking to diversify into health care, as well as into household commodities and clothing. Asda has begun offering flu jabs for shoppers, at a cost of £11.97 per jab – a great deal less than the £20 typically charged by GPs for a private jab. Asda's service appeals mainly to the 'worried well', as those for whom the flu jab is clinically indicated get it free through the NHS.[39] But this initiative seems likely to be only a starter. U First Healthcare has identified 250 Tesco stores as potential sites for setting up GP practices and has opened pilot surgeries in some of them. U First Healthcare already has surgeries in hotels such as the Marriott at Manchester airport, besides running surgeries elsewhere for which patients pay £150 a year for membership, and £50 per twenty-minute consultation.[40]

Other mainstream retail companies, including Boots and Superdrug, are also making forays into primary health care provision. Boots has incorporated Medicentre-branded surgeries into several of its shops. This US concept is also the model for the NHS walk-in centres, and Boots also hosts one of these, blurring the boundary between the NHS and the private sector in another way. Birmingham's NHS walk-in centre was opened in Boots's city centre store in March 2000. A team of thirteen nurses, supported by healthcare assistants and voluntary sector advisers, provides advice on minor illnesses, basic blood pressure and urine testing, and health information. It is not difficult to envisage this whole operation being transferred to the private sector under the new GP contract.

Boots is positioning itself to take a greater share of NHS business. As well as offering travel and health care insurance it has introduced in-store podiatry services and in 1999 it launched six dental practices. It is also now providing routine NHS cataract eye surgery and some lens surgery currently not available on the NHS.

Nursing home chains integrating with primary care

As we saw in Chapter 1, Westminster Health Care is currently the third-largest nursing and residential care provider in the UK. It also offers several integrated health care packages in primary care centres, subacute hospitals, intermediate care, and town hospitals for populations of 50,000–100,000. Its stated aim is to 'bring together private sector expertise in business management and finance with those professionals responsible for the delivery of care on the ground'.[41] Some general practitioners are now practising in the company's private hospitals or renting space from the company for NHS care.

OPENING UP GENERAL PRACTICE PREMISES TO THE PRIVATE SECTOR

Even though since 1966 GPs had been partially reimbursed for their investment in practice premises, via the General Practice Finance Corporation, many GPs, especially in deprived areas, were often still practising from their homes, with inadequate space and facilities. By the 1990s, too, GPs increasingly needed to provide accommodation for nurse-run specialist clinics, as more and more services were transferred from hospitals to primary care. After 1997 the new flexibility offered by the PMS contract created opportunities for alternative models of ownership of primary care facilities, accelerating the existing trend towards for-profit organisations purchasing GP premises and even employing GPs.[42] Moreover in 1989 the Conservative government had sold the General Practice Finance Corporation (GPFC), which provided loans to GPs for practice premises, to Norwich Union Life Insurance Society for £145 million. This meant that private corporations could now invest in NHS primary care and secure repayment out of NHS revenues.

In 2001 the Labour government proposed to take these developments further by extending the PFI idea to primary care in the shape of a new Local Improvement Finance Trust (LIFT), which would set up local subsidiaries or joint ventures with private companies. The government proposed an investment of £1 billion to refurbish 3,000 GP premises and to build 500 'one-stop' health centres, where patients could receive care not only from their GP but also from professionals such as pharmacists, physiotherapists and podiatrists.[43] This initiative was partly influenced by the requirements of the 1995 Disability Discrimination Act, under which all existing premises had to be made fully accessible to disabled people by October 2004.

Local LIFT companies can purchase, develop and sell land, and establish subsidiaries to generate income in joint undertakings with other parties. GPs and other potential occupants of the premises such as pharmacists and dentists can lease space directly from the local LIFT company, or indirectly via their PCT. Unlike traditional leases, the LIFT company will be responsible for the maintenance, repair and insurance of the property.

At first sight, LIFT appears attractive to GPs, and particularly to the many who wish to practise in deprived areas but without the risks involved in owning property in them. Previously their main alternative had been to sign long leases, which were restrictive in nature and under which they were also responsible for property maintenance. LIFT started operating in six inner-city areas in 2001, including Newcastle and Manchester; by 2003 there were forty-two LIFT schemes. In Nottingham four PCTs joined together in a scheme estimated to cost £123 million to overhaul all the primary care premises in the city.

Despite many reservations on the part of GPs, LIFT now often appears to be the only way available to improve their premises. As Dr Chris Locke, the Secretary of Nottingham Local Medical Committee, put it: 'some people do have problems with the involvement of the private sector but the fact is that this is the only show in town. If it delivers the goods, then so be it. It is the only way we can solve all the difficulties with premises'.[44]

The extent to which LIFT and private finance are changing the ownership of primary care premises and channelling more NHS revenues into corporate hands is not yet widely appreciated. In 2000, primary care services were provided by 29,987 general practitioners in 9,000 main surgeries and 2,500 branch surgeries. The most recent survey of ownership carried out by the NHS Executive's valuation office in 1995-96 showed that 63 per cent of practice premises were owned by general practitioners, 16 per cent were owned by the NHS, and 21 per cent were rented from the private sector.[45] Now, however, health care companies, property companies and multinational conglomerates with health care interests are increasingly assuming ownership of primary care facilities.

There are currently around eight market leaders engaged in negotiating more than 300 projects on GP premises. They include Primary Health Properties, Primary Health Care Centres, the GP Investment Corporation, and Primary Medical Properties. Some are subsidiaries of larger groups. One is Sinclair Montrose's Healthcare Property company, while another is Primary Medical Properties, an operating division of the building contractor Morgan Sindall. The GP Investment Corporation is part of the GP Group, a holding company for various investments in property, transport, and health care. Others, such as Primary Health Care Centres, are freestanding concerns. Primary Health Properties, although nominally an independent company with its own shareholders, has its portfolio managed by Nexus Management Services, part of the larger Nexus group. Nexus is a financial advisory company that is currently establishing partnership arrangements with several primary care groups and trusts.

Property companies are also increasingly diversifying into both non-clinical and clinical operations. In January 2000, the *Sunday Times* reported that Topland was planning to become Britain's biggest owner of doctors' surgeries. The company's owners, the Zakay brothers, had set aside £100 million of their family fortune to invest in the sector. Topland plans to buy the surgeries and lease them back to GPs at agreed rents, which will then effectively be underwritten by the government. Topland has modelled its business on Rotch, a larger private property company, which is currently involved in several private finance initiative and public–private partnership projects in the health sector. These include complex 'bundlings' of community, hospital and mental health facilities, such as the Queen Mary's Sidcup NHS Trusts, Oxleas NHS Trust, and Sedgefield Community Hospital.

Even more ambitious projects involving the privatisation of NHS premises are being developed by Norwich Union (the owners since 1989 of the General Practice Finance Corporation, as noted above).

Bradford Community Trust, for example, has signed a £4 million deal with Norwich Union on behalf of the Horton Park Medical Centre in West Yorkshire, which will include three general practices, a pharmacy, an optician, a restaurant, and a welfare benefits office. The Sedgley Community Health Centre in the West Midlands is a £3.5 million joint venture between Norwich Union and health and local authorities to provide purpose-built integrated care facilities for use by social workers, visiting nurses, and a general practitioner 'out of hours' service. It will also provide dental and family planning services, a library, a base for the local mental health team, and offices for Age Concern and the Citizens' Advice Bureau. Norwich Union will get access to patients and doctors for marketing its private health care and health insurance products, in addition to the secure revenue flows from the NHS budget that lease-holders will provide, plus the potentially significant degree of influence over future clinical developments that ownership of the premises confers.

For as occupants of corporate-owned premises GPs will have less power to alter or develop their practices than they have as owner occu-piers, since they will need to seek approval from the company for alterations. Moreover the details of the contracts with the property companies, and the repayment schedules, are not in the public domain, so there has been no thorough independent evaluation of the revenue implications. In the longer run patients may not prove to be well served by the resulting transfer of power away from GP practices, where there is professional accountability, to property corporations. Health needs and priorities could become secondary to the interests of shareholders.

Alternative models for financing and funding practices do exist. Aside from the option of publicly owned premises, the BMA has proposed grants to help GPs avoid negative equity by guaranteeing minimum sale prices for their premises, and grants to restore premises to residential use if they come to be deemed unsuitable for use as a surgery. Instead the LIFT scheme and private finance not only encourage the private sector to become key players in the ownership of premises but also move closer to making primary care subject to corporate agendas, with seem-ingly little or no evaluation of the implications for equity or efficiency in the provision of primary health care.[46]

ACCOUNTABILITY AND REGULATION OF PRIMARY CARE

Of the three big scandals in recent years that have served to reshape the regulation of the medical profession, the case of serial killer Dr Harold Shipman, a Manchester GP, played an extraordinary role in reshaping general practice: as one Department of Health official commented, Shipman allowed the government to impose changes that the General Medical Council (GMC) would never previously have accepted.

Since 1858 the medical profession had been allowed largely to regulate itself. In order to practise, doctors had to register with the GMC and thereafter only came under professional scrutiny if they were reported for unethical or incompetent practice. GPs could also be disciplined for any breaches in the terms and conditions of their contract, but this primarily covered practice administration and finance rather than clinical practice. Now the medical profession was to become far more accountable to the state.

As a result of the political pressure for change, the GMC instituted a radical reform, requiring the revalidation of every registered doctor. In order to be able to keep their licences to practise, every five years all registered doctors now have to submit to the GMC evidence that their practice is satisfactory. New measures for the closer monitoring of GPs, especially single-handed practitioners, were also included in the Health and Social Care Bill of 2003 because, the government said, 'although most single-handed GPs work hard and are committed to their patients, they tend to operate in relative clinical isolation'.[47] Health authorities were required to hold lists of all GPs in their areas and were given new powers to suspend, remove, or refuse to admit GPs on to their lists on grounds of inefficiency, fraud or unsuitability. GPs sentenced to more than six months in prison had to be removed from the list.

These regulatory reforms, especially those targeting single-handed GPs, were to tie in with the changes under the 2002 GP contract. At the same time new arrangements were also put in place to make PCTs themselves more accountable for operationalising the market.

Each of the 303 PCTs in England is monitored by one of the twenty-eight strategic health authorities, and is required to provide the public with independently validated Patient Prospectuses, published annually, giving information about the availability and performance of the local health service. The Commission for Healthcare Audit and Inspection (CHAI) will also have an important new role in primary care, as the inspector of both public and private health care providers. Another far-reaching change in terms of accountability and regulation is the 2003 Health and Social Care Act which allows high-performing or three-star NHS trusts to apply for foundation status, with all the powers that go with it. If PCTs can get foundation status, as the White Paper *Delivering the NHS Plan* proposed, they can in effect float themselves off as not-for-profit companies which, like hospital foundation trusts, will come under the independent regulator who then will be the decisive influence in determining what services a PCT provides, and how.[48] In approving a PCT's licence the independent regulator will take into account the existing market for services in the area. This could mean that some foundation PCTs will not be licensed to provide some elements of primary care, and that in turn would mean that the GP practices within that PCT would have even less say about what care they delivered.

THE EMERGING 'MIXED ECONOMY' OF PRIMARY CARE

In 2003 most PCTs were still struggling to define their organisational role. Like the hospital trusts before them, they were too numerous and therefore too small to be able to employ many staff with a strategic vision, and turned instead to costly external consultants and temporary staff as they grappled with the finance, commissioning, public health and primary care issues on their agendas. PCTs and general practices were brought somewhat closer together as they tried to assume their new roles, though the extent to which this was true varied considerably from place to place. What was certainly true was that through the PCTs, supervised by the strategic health authorities, the culture of 'star ratings' and 'performance management' was increasingly influencing decision-making in primary care; the principle of planning primary services based on population needs was being increasingly eclipsed, and the amount of effective attention devoted to the integration of the increasingly fragmented primary care services, and the integration of primary care with hospital care, was to say the least limited.

The immediate issue was how PCTs would manage the implementation of the new GP contract due to come into force in April 2004. For the first time PCTs would be fully responsible for primary care, and would have to deal with commissioning it from other providers than GPs, or even have to provide some elements of it themselves, if GP practices decided to withdraw from the provision of non-'essential' services. There were reports that eight out of ten GPs planned to opt out of providing care at night and weekends.[49]

The renegotiation of contracts for pharmacists and terms of service for other health care professionals such as nurses does have a potential to produce more flexibility in the delivery of primary care, but it is a central part of New Labour's plan to introduce a 'mixed economy' of primary care providers, moving away from a GP-led service. But this will clearly be at the expense of the continuity of care provided by traditional British general practice, which is valued by patients and admired worldwide. As with GP fundholding, there is also a potential for high transaction costs, and for widening inequities in access and in the quality of primary care. If the experience of the PFI in hospital building, the higher 'tariff' that will be paid to private providers of DTCs or ITCs, and the new revenue claims of LIFT schemes, are any guide, this will mean that significant amounts of local NHS revenue are diverted to provide profits for the private sector.

Above all, the new 'mixed economy' in primary care will change incentives. There will be a growing range of alternative health care providers, with whom GPs will have to compete for supplying different elements of care. As a result GPs may, willingly or not, begin selecting on financial grounds the types of service they wish to provide, and who they wish to provide them to – in effect, cherry-picking or cream-skimming – with the result that the less attractive services are provided more cheaply by others, at lower levels of quality. Experience from the USA shows that devolving financial risk downwards will result in practices seeking to minimise it. Groups such as the homeless, the chronically sick and asylum seekers may find it even harder than at present to obtain access to care. The focus on performance payments also gives GPs an incentive to cherry-pick the patients and the services they provide.[50]

All this is necessarily speculation, but as this book was going to press the logic involved was strikingly confirmed when the government announced that from 1 April 2004 it was lifting the ban introduced in 1948 (see page 129) on the sale of 'goodwill' in the provision of non-'essential' GP services, such as out of hours cover, immunisations, etc. In this instance the commercial value of goodwill will be linked to the types of patients and their likelihood of enabling the service provider to meet government performance targets. Allowing the providers of non-'essential' primary care services – who can include GPs – to include goodwill when selling their businesses effectively endorses the operation of primary care services for profit. Indeed, the government's explicit aim was to encourage competition between GPs and private firms.

Although 'essential' GP services are supposed to be excluded, in practice this distinction will be hard to draw. If GPs choose to provide non-'essential' services themselves they will have an incentive to select patients so as to increase the profitability of doing so. A private company providing these services will have an incentive to work up a profitable business and then sell it, with obvious costs in terms of continuity and quality of care. The new policy was imposed over the objections of the BMA's GPs Committee.

The private sector has now secured the foothold it wanted and it is not hard to predict what will happen. In some of the prosperous areas which formerly had a high proportion of fundholders, PCTs will become powerful, competing with hospitals to develop rival health care 'products'. But the general model will be one dominated by private companies, which either buy GPs out and put them on a salary, or retire them. The large number of GPs who are approaching retirement tired and disillusioned are resigned to the future: for them, the question is how much they can get for selling their share in the practice. Incoming GPs will not be able to compete with the commercial sector in the scramble for lucrative practices, especially in the prosperous shires. General practices that don't move in this direction could find themselves struggling to keep patients and income, and with premises that have little commercial value.

The last obstacles to the entry of the private sector into primary care have thus now been removed. First, the use of private finance for the infrastructure (LIFT) has facilitated the transfer of ownership from GPs to corporations. Next, the renegotiation of the GP contract and remuneration of GP services means that services are being broken up and put into the marketplace. Finally, the reintroduction of the sale of 'goodwill' enables primary care to be made profitable by having profitable patients – i.e. potential customers for private health insurance and private health care, or patients who are selected for their low risk to the practice and the likelihood that they will make it easy for the practice to achieve the government targets that trigger additional payments. In Australia, corporations have been able to purchase a growing proportion of general practices and convert the GPs in them into salaried company staff, maximising profits by selecting patients for their profitability and referring them for pathology and other services also provided by the corporation. As and when PCTs start to become foundation trusts, free to enter into joint ventures with private companies and to look for new sources of income, there seems no obvious reason why this will not happen in Britain too. This is the market that the UnitedHealth Group intends to target.[51]

6

LONG-TERM CARE FOR OLDER PEOPLE

Of all the areas of social policy, long-term care for older people is perhaps the most riddled with inequities and injustices. Unlike hospital care and education, which are organised and funded on collective principles, primary responsibility for the care of frail older people is not borne by the state but is largely left to relatives and friends who care for them in their own homes. This largely invisible workforce amounts to some 5.7 million people providing care to older people. About 800,000 of them are providing unpaid care for fifty hours a week or more.[1] The burden falls disproportionately on the poorer and older members of society; indeed many of those providing care are in need of care themselves.[2]

When the state does intervene it is mainly when this informal network is unable to cope. But rather than provide care directly, the state has now largely turned long-term care over to private enterprise, and over the past two decades has created a for-profit industry worth some £6.9 billion a year.[3] In 2003, 90 per cent of nursing home beds and 63 per cent of residential care beds for elderly, chronically ill and physically disabled people in the UK were operated on a for-profit basis.[4] The almost 400,000 older people in these homes are now a source of income and profit for an increasingly corporatised sector.[5]

While for most care home residents the cost of care is in practice covered by the state through local authority funding, in England and Wales free long-term care is no longer a right, and over the past fifteen to twenty years the NHS has almost totally withdrawn from the provision of long-term care. The result is that many thousands of older people who had once been promised free care in their final years are now paying for it. Before the state will meet the cost, people must demonstrate that they are too poor to pay. For those who do pay, charges are levied on some kinds of care that used to be considered part of the free care offered by the NHS.

And despite having to pay for their health care, most care home residents receive 'haphazard' services. According to the Royal College of Physicians, the Royal College of Nursing and the British Geriatric Society, most medical staff with responsibility for care homes do not have specialist training, with the result that vulnerable residents with complex health problems are not getting services tailored to their needs. Up to one-quarter of residents receive inappropriate medication, and the services provided by chiropodists, optometrists and psychiatric nurses are inconsistent.[6] Moreover, while the general public receive free treatment from their GPs, many thousands of care home residents are being charged over £40 a year for GP services.[7]

This erosion of collective responsibility has not gone unchallenged. Pensioner groups and organisations representing older people have accused successive governments of betraying the 1948 promise of 'cradle to grave' care. Indeed a strong sense that the social contract was being broken in this respect led the incoming Labour government in 1997 to set up a Royal Commission to examine the funding of long-term care. But although the Royal Commission reported in 1999, reaffirming the 1948 consensus that long-term care should be a collective responsibility, the Labour government rejected its findings; the Prime Minister declared that the 'money would be better spent elsewhere'.[8] By 2000 the Treasury and the Department of Health were wedded to market solutions and the long-term care industry had become too powerful to challenge.

PENALISED FOR LIVING LONGER?

That health care services for older people have been subject to cutbacks and privatisation over the past two decades should perhaps come as no surprise, since older people as a group often find themselves at the margins of modern-day society. Almost one-quarter of all pensioners in the UK live below the poverty line.[9] Assigned the status of 'dependants', many older people are unable to participate fully in society, and many are subject to discrimination and unreported abuse. Their detachment from the rest of society is commonly regarded as a natural result of ageing, but in fact the vast majority of people over sixty-five are fit and healthy and able to look after themselves; two-thirds of those over seventy-five have no physical difficulty undertaking ordinary daily activities, and the proportion of people over sixty-five who live in care homes is a mere 5 per cent.[10] Older people do consume more health care than younger people, but this is mainly because most health care expenditure takes place within the last year of life, as is equally true for people of all ages.[11]

Yet because most older people are no longer 'economically' productive, the common perception of older people is that they are a burden on the resources of the state and the working population. In this sense policy-makers are still influenced by an idea openly stated by a royal commission on population over fifty years ago: 'the old consume without producing, which differentiates them from the active population and makes them a factor reducing the average standard of living of the community'.[12]

This image of older people as a burden on the rest of society has been enforced in recent years by scare stories about the 'demographic time bomb' – the idea that as people live longer, welfare systems are no longer sustainable. The ageing of societies throughout the world clearly does have implications for state-funded welfare programmes. As people live longer there are greater demands on the health care system and greater reliance on savings and pensions, while the declining ratio of workers to non-workers threatens to lead to a reduction in the overall resources available. But the facts do not support the alarmism spread by policy-makers and government ministers on this score. Improvements in medical technology, a decrease in the number of dependent children, and a healthier older workforce willing to continue to participate in the labour market will all ameliorate the 'negative' effects of an ageing Britain.[13] The neo-liberal response of welfare cutbacks and privatisation is thus an ideological position unsupported by sound analysis or evidence. In many ways it is a throwback to the philosophy of the Poor Laws, according to which individuals were responsible for their own welfare, and institutional care was only for the 'deserving poor' and so was only provided following a stigmatising test of needs and means. Although the twentieth century saw massive advances in technology and huge increases in the overall standard of living, this attitude still prevails: we still see fit to force some 70,000 old people every year to sell their homes and pay most of the proceeds in fees before they can receive state-funded residential care.[14]

LONG-TERM CARE BEFORE THATCHER

Many of the current problems in long-term care provision for older people have historical roots in the post-Second World War welfare settlement. Although charging for care services has only become commonplace over the past two decades, the principle of charging was established as long ago as 1948. Moreover such long-term care provision as has been provided has always been undertaken by voluntary or private agencies as well as the state, a fact that undoubtedly made it easier for neo-liberal policy-makers to reduce the role of the state in this area from the 1980s onwards.

Of course, none of today's developments were inevitable. Indeed the immediate post-1945 period promised better and more equitable treatment for sick older people than anything that had gone before. The much-reviled Poor Laws were abolished and two welfare reform acts, the 1946 NHS Act and the 1948 National Assistance Act, were introduced. Between them, these reforms promised that the state would provide universal health care for all, a right of citizens irrespective of age or ability to pay. But the two pieces of legislation established two parallel systems of care. The NHS would provide a universal system of health care organised along collective principles and free at the point of delivery, while under the National Assistance Act local authorities would provide a subsidiary system for those in need of other 'care and attention'. The care to be provided by local authorities was primarily concerned with frail older people, but unlike NHS care it was means-tested and subject to a statutory charge.

In making a distinction between those people who were 'sick' and those who were in need of 'care and attention' the architects of the welfare state introduced a fault line which would later be exploited by governments from Thatcher onwards. In particular, the definition of what conditions need 'care and attention' would be expanded to include a range of chronic sicknesses, in relation to which care could then be charged for. Aneurin Bevan, who had introduced the distinction, had had a quite different intention. He meant the National Assistance Act to provide care for 'the type of old person who is still able to look after themselves but who is unable to do the housework, the laundry, cook meals and things of that sort' (i.e. people who needed domestic help) – a very different type of person from most of those currently living in Britain's care homes, whose health care needs are very considerable.[15]

The post-war Labour government wanted to construct the kind of residential care homes for older people that had previously been the preserve of the rich. As Bevan told parliament, 'the whole idea is that welfare authorities should provide them and charge an economic rent for them so that any old persons who wish to go may go there in exactly the same way as many well to do people have been accustomed to go into residential hotels'.[16] It should be noted that this vision of local authority provision did not include other kinds of community-based state provision, such as domiciliary care (i.e. services provided in people's own homes), yet it was a bold vision, especially given the resource constraints of the immediate post-war years, since it implied a major expansion in the number of 'hotel-style' care homes.

Until this could happen the government relied on the voluntary sector – organisations such as the Salvation Army, Cheshire Homes, Darby and Joan Homes, Cross Roads, Marie Curie, the Church Army, the Methodists and others – to provide not only residential homes but also community-based services. From 1948 onwards this 'third sector' played a major role in long-term care provision; in 1972 it was still providing 18 per cent of all residential care for older people.[17] Initially, the state was even more dependent on the voluntary sector to provide care services to the many older people who were fit enough to remain in their own homes but needed help with their meals and laundry, or who sought companionship in local lunch and recreation clubs. While the 1946 National Health Service Act gave local health authorities the power to develop these services, it did not give them the power to provide them directly. Instead the Ministry of Health urged local authorities to do 'everything in their power to encourage further voluntary effort to meet the needs of old people.'[18]

But while the voluntary sector remained a significant force in the provision of residential care it was not large or co-ordinated enough to take on the responsibility for providing domiciliary services on an adequate scale. So when the importance of community-based provision began to be more fully recognised – in the main because of concern over the high cost of residential care – the state was forced to step in. Legislation was passed in the late 1960s allowing local authorities to provide domiciliary care services themselves; the state then became the dominant provider and remained so until the end of the 1990s. In 1992 only 2 per cent of home-care hours funded by local authorities were provided by non-profit voluntary or private for-profit providers.[19]

UNDERMINING THE POST-WAR SETTLEMENT

While the dual system described above later permitted a significant curtailment of free health care, the system put in place by Bevan was free from many of today's inequities. The intention was that older people would have most of their health care needs met in hospital free of charge but would pay, where they could, for accommodation and assistance in 'hotel-style' rest homes if they needed full-time care but not hospitalisation.

But Bevan's plan for local authority homes to be like hotels, looking after people who were merely frail, rather than sick or infirm, failed to materialise. By 1965 the Ministry of Health was telling local authorities that they were expected to take on responsibility for

> ... residents who fall ill, whether for short or long periods, [but] whose needs are no greater than could be met in their own homes by relatives with the aid of the local health services. Where the illness is expected to be terminal transfer to hospital should be avoided unless continuous medical or nursing care is necessary. Some incontinent residents (other than those with intractable incontinence and other disabilities) may also be manageable in a residential home.[20]

So local authorities increasingly assumed responsibility for caring for more and more heavily dependent people in care homes. One London borough council which sought help from the health service in the mid-1970s over the increased dependency of its care home residents was informed by the local health authority that there was a failure to grasp the changing notion of nursing care.[21] This came following a review of the older people living in its ten residential care homes which revealed that one in five needed help moving between rooms and one in nine was doubly incontinent, that significant numbers were either somewhat or severely confused, and that considerable staff time was being consumed in overseeing the taking of drugs and providing basic nursing care.[22]

Not only were local authority care home staff having to deal with much sicker individuals but more and more older people found themselves being treated not in NHS hospitals, where health care was free, but instead within a means-tested system of long-term care where charges could be levied. The state also failed to provide the necessary expansion or upgrading of long-term care facilities. As in other areas of state expenditure, 'unproductive' older people were at the back of the queue when resources were distributed. By 1954 only forty-three new buildings had been provided nationwide, while 755 existing premises had been converted.[23] It was not until 1960 that the number of new residential care homes built exceeded thirty a year.[24]

The inability or unwillingness of governments to devote capital resources to the construction of high-quality long-term care facilities has been a constant theme in the history of the welfare state since 1945, and was one of the main reasons why private capital was so easily introduced into the provision of institutional care for older people in the last two decades of the twentieth century. The lack of investment in care homes for older people, as well as the failure to provide domiciliary care services, left many older people, even in the late 1970s, residing in poorly-converted workhouses.[25]

LONG-TERM CARE UNDER THATCHER AND MAJOR

Cutting back on state provision for older people and the creation of the for-profit sector

The 'mixed economy' of long-term care created by this history of state parsimony made long-term care particularly vulnerable to attack by the New Right, and particularly susceptible to their neo-liberal policies, as Drakeford points out in relation to social services generally:

> The mixed pattern of provision struck two important chords with the incoming administration of 1979. On the one hand, it suggested that – unlike education or health, for example – the social services provided promising territory for increased private sector involvement and the promotion of a market in social care. On the other, it chimed with an even more fundamental Conservative instinct that the primary responsibility for care of this sort should lie, not with the state at all, but with families and charitable provision.[26]

Moreover since the 1950s a consensus had developed about the desirability of 'community care': the idea that where older people needed to be cared for by the state, it should where possible be in their own homes and not in large impersonal institutions. This consensus too was exploited by the New Right. By appealing to the ideas of many academics and commentators on the benefits of 'care in the community' the Thatcher and Major governments were able to enlist the support of many of the key stakeholders for their agenda.[27] But the Conservative conception of 'community care' was in reality very different from what most people had understood by de-institutionalisation. The purpose of the Thatcher and Major reforms was both to eliminate almost entirely the role of the state in the provision of services for older people and to reduce to a minimum its responsibility for funding them. The aim was to stimulate an active market in the provision of care services (which would in turn produce the 'efficiency savings' that are supposed to flow from market competition), and to transfer the costs of funding care in old age to individuals and their families.

But before such a market could be created, private providers needed to be certain that the state would underwrite the risks involved; before private financiers would support any investment in care homes or other support services a guaranteed income stream was necessary. This was first provided from the government's centrally administered social security budget, and later from its budgetary allocations to local authorities.

The first Thatcher government began its assault on the state provision of care for the elderly almost as soon as it entered office by sharply reducing the funding of local authority social services departments.[28] This meant that the income of the voluntary organisations on whose care homes local authorities depended began to dry up. In 1974 local authorities had paid for almost 60 per cent of voluntary sector care home residents in England; by 1983 the proportion was down to 34 per cent.[29] With funding from local authorities in short supply, the voluntary care home sector was kept afloat by the social security benefits received by those residents who were unable to pay their own fees, and for whom local authorities were unable or unwilling to pay the full amount. In effect, Department of Social Security officers started to pay an income-related benefit (now known as Income Support) to residents in voluntary sector care homes to enable them to pay the fees.

Although this practice began here and there at the local level, it quickly became widespread and by 1983 had developed into a formal system for funding care for older people in 'independent-sector' – i.e. non–local-authority – homes. As well as reducing the pressure on local authority budgets the new funding system also ushered in an era of consumer choice, since it allowed poorer people to choose a care home in the voluntary or private sector with the Department of Social Security footing the bill. And unlike for those who entered local authority homes there was no assessment of the patient's actual need for care services. Moreover, since money came out of open-ended national social security expenditure, it was not subject to the same constraints as overstretched and cash-limited local authority budgets.

This created a new opportunity for private entrepreneurs. With access to flexible sources of private investment, as well as business start-up grants provided by the government, for-profit care homes began to spring up around the country. A rapid expansion of private residential and nursing care began.[30]

But local authorities remained starved of cash, and because the Department of Social Security (DSS) would only fund people in voluntary or for-profit homes, many local authorities started to cut back on their own provision of care home places in the knowledge that the DSS and the private sector would fill the gap. Thus between 1982 and 1992 the number of residents in local authority residential homes fell by nearly one-third.[31] The same thing happened in the NHS, as Figure 6.1 shows. The new availability of funds from the social security budget for 'independent' care homes allowed the NHS to discharge dependent patients from long-term care hospital wards into private residential care.[32]

Major corporate providers – as opposed to the typical small-scale private owner with one or at most two homes – also began to be attracted into the care home market by the scale of the new funding from the social security budget. But the cost of 'pump priming' a new care home market in this way was considerable. In 1979 there were some 11,000 recipients of Income Support in private and voluntary nursing and residential homes, at an annual cost to the DSS of £10 million. By 1990 there were 281,200 such recipients and the annual cost had risen to £2.6 billion.[33]

Despite concerns about the rising cost of the social security budget the policy allowed the Conservatives to achieve their two main goals: downsizing local authority and NHS provision and promoting the private sector. And the speed at which the private, for-profit sector moved into a dominant market position was astonishing. In 1979, 16 per cent of residential care homes were in the for-profit sector and 20 per cent in the voluntary (not-for-profit) sector. By April 2003, of the national total of 501,900 places available for long-term care of the elderly and physically disabled, 346,100 (69 per cent) were in the for-profit sector and 71,000 (14 per cent) in the voluntary sector. Just 17 per cent remained in the public sector (i.e. run by the NHS or local authorities).[34]

The massive growth of the for-profit care home sector was often damaging to the interests of many older people. Because it was essentially 'free' for local authorities to place an older person in a private care home, they tended to place them in care homes rather than provide domiciliary care or other support services which would have allowed them to maintain independent lives. According to Gerald Wistow, by 1991 27 per cent more people had been moved into care homes than would have been the case if the 1981 balance between domiciliary care

Figure 6.1 The switch from state to private provision of long-term care for older people in the UK

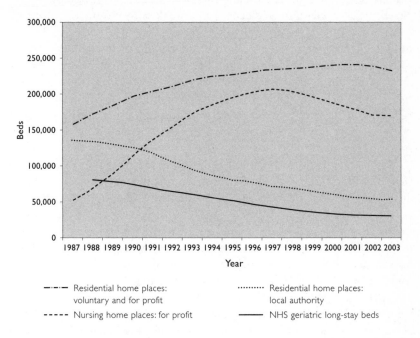

Source: Laing and Buisson, *Care of Elderly People Market Survey 2003*, London 2003, p. 26, Table 2.2

and care home admission had been retained; and the provision of home help and 'meals on wheels' for people aged seventy-five and over fell by 15 per cent and 14 per cent respectively between 1977/78 and 1984/85, and by a further 10 and 13 per cent respectively between 1986/87 and 1992/93.[35] Older people who could have been looked after in their own homes paid a high price for the establishment of the multibillion-pound care home market.

Increasing concerns over the rising social security bill, and a report by the Audit Commission in 1986 criticising the perverse incentives against providing domiciliary care led the Thatcher government to ask

Sir Roy Griffiths (who as we saw in Chapter 3 had reported on hospital management in 1983) to review the funding of community care.[36] But the 1988 Griffiths report, and the 1990 NHS and Community Care Act that followed it, simply accelerated market developments. Griffiths recommended that local authorities should take over responsibility for funding all long-term care from the Department of Social Security, but move away from providing care themselves to being purchasers of services within a 'mixed economy' of care.[37] In this way local authorities would be compelled to control expenditure both through the rationing of services to older people and through using their purchasing power as bulk buyers to drive down the prices charged by private care home operators.[38]

While some local authorities liked their new role as purchasers rather than providers, others had to be forced into it through the use of financial incentives. After 1993, councils had to fund all community care out of the Personal Social Services (PSS) allocation in the annual block grants they received from central government. In order to soften the impact of this new burden a Special Transition Grant (STG) was added, but 85 per cent of this grant had to be spent on care provided by the 'independent sector'. The STG was a substantial part of the PSS allocation from central government, so the new arrangements effectively forced local authorities to contract out the provision of care. Local authorities were further locked into using the market by the fact that the 1990 NHS and Community Care Act also required them to take over the funding of nursing care provision for people in care homes. Contracting with the independent sector thus became the dominant method of delivering care services.

The government even gave local authorities a further financial incentive to place older people in need in independent sector care homes by allowing the local authorities to recoup part of their residents' Income Support benefit known as 'residential allowance'. Since local authorities were only able to access this source of income for residents in independent sector homes this provided a very significant incentive to place older people in independent sector residential care. In effect, in 2000, for every resident who was placed in an independent sector home (and was entitled to the benefit), the local authority was able to recoup £61.80 a week.

These financial incentives also led many local authorities to transfer or sell their own existing care homes to the independent sector. A House of Lords ruling in 1996 found that local authorities could fulfil their duties under the 1948 National Assistance Act without providing services directly.[39] This meant that they did not need to retain their care homes, and so, in what was probably one of the most under-reported sell-offs of the Thatcher and Major years, hundreds of care homes and the land attached to them were transferred to for-profit companies or voluntary associations at rock-bottom prices. In Scotland, for example, Dumfries and Galloway Council obtained consent from the government to sell five residential care homes with a total market value of £2.03 million to a private company for £1 each.[40] A study conducted in 1996 found that over 12 per cent of all independent residential care homes had been purchased or transferred from local authorities, and given the large number of transfers that have taken place since then, the percentage is now probably much higher.[41] Not only was the state guaranteeing mainly for-profit providers an income stream from the public purse, it was also transferring to them, at little or even no cost, substantial assets that had been paid for out of public funds.

Free health care for all? – again

The creation of a market in long-term care was only part of the New Right's health care agenda. Cash-strapped local authorities had to ration and charge for care which meant that individuals and their families took on an increased financial burden. The role of the unpaid 'informal sector' was formalised in the government's 1989 White Paper *Caring for People*, which recognised that relatives, friends and neighbours provided most of the care for frail older people.[42] It was, however, clearly the government's intention that things should stay that way. Social security benefits were provided to assist carers at home, but they were far from adequate to meet the true costs or to compensate them for the loss of earnings and isolation from the community that their work entailed.[43] Disability pressure groups had campaigned for care *in* the community, that is, state-funded care outside of large institutions, but the Conservatives' agenda meant care *by* the community – or, rather, by unpaid family members and friends.

The NHS also participated in this process of passing the buck. Between 1976 and 1994 the number of NHS beds specifically designated for older people fell from 56,000 to 37,500, a reduction of 33 per cent.[44] While the closing of outdated geriatric and psychogeriatric facilities was long overdue, terminating NHS provision meant that costs were transferred to individuals on a dramatic scale as increasing numbers of people who would formerly have been NHS patients and cared for free of charge now entered a means-tested system. The exact number of older people in today's nursing homes who would have received free NHS care in the past is impossible to know. But the level of ill-health among many nursing home patients suggested to the House of Commons Health Select Committee in 1995 that the numbers were indeed significant.[45]

The extent to which the NHS had withdrawn from caring for the long-term sick only really became apparent in 1994 when the Health Ombudsman upheld a complaint against a Leeds hospital that had discharged a doubly incontinent, brain-damaged 55-year-old man, who could not feed himself, to a private nursing home, on the grounds that it could not improve his condition.[46] By discharging the man into local authority care the hospital transferred the cost of his care to the man's wife. The case raised the question of the ability of the NHS to refuse to accept responsibility for such a clearly sick individual. The government responded by, in effect, introducing eligibility criteria for free NHS care. The Department of Health now ruled that only people with 'complex or multiple healthcare needs' that required 'continuing and specialist medical or nursing supervision' had the right to free NHS care.[47]

And while the NHS was offloading the costs of sick and frail older people onto individuals and their families, local authorities were coming under increased pressure to ration and charge for their services. This stemmed partly from the fact that under the 1990 NHS and Community Care Act local authorities were being asked to take on responsibility for funding both residential and nursing care for older people, a cost that had previously been met from the social security budget. Yet local authorities were finding it increasingly difficult to pay for this out of their cash-limited Community Care budgets. In 1996 a report by the Association of County Councils found that local authorities were spending around 7 per cent above their budgets for social services and concluded that £116 million would have to be cut from local authority spending on community care services in order to balance the books.[48] Most local authorities began ranking people in terms of their 'assessed needs' and providing care only for the most dependent. Some departments set ceilings on costs, while others operated waiting lists.[49] In the case of frail older people who were declared ineligible for support, the burden was simply left with relatives, friends and neighbours.

The budgetary pressure placed on local authorities by the transfer of responsibilities under the 1990 Act meant that they were more likely to levy charges on individuals for all services, including domiciliary care. Although during the 1980s local authorities had been given discretionary power to charge for domiciliary services, most of them had resisted this pressure, and charging even declined over this period.[50] But from the early 1990s onwards this changed dramatically. Despite the fact that local authorities' charging powers still remained discretionary, central government allocated resources to local authorities on the assumption that 9 per cent of the costs of domiciliary services would be recovered through charges. Altogether some £260 million was cut from the allocations to local authorities nationwide, and many local authorities were left with no choice but to charge for domiciliary care. As the Local Government Anti-Poverty Unit put it: 'The extent to which people on low incomes will be protected will depend upon the extent to which the authority forgoes potential income.'[51] By 2000, 94 per cent of councils were charging for domiciliary or home care services, compared with only 72 per cent in 1992/93.[52]

There is no national means test for domiciliary care services, and so local authorities have been free to determine their own local policies. This has led to a highly inequitable situation. People in similar circumstances but living in different areas face charges for domiciliary services that vary from nothing to well over £100 per week for the same level of service. Moreover, while nearly two-thirds of councils exempt those on the lowest incomes from charges, over one-third charge people who are in receipt of Income Support, leaving them with less to live on than the Income Support amount appropriate to their age.[53]

The squeezing of community care budgets also made local authorities more likely to pursue those who were deemed able to pay for residential care. According to the poverty expert Saul Becker, social services departments started to tighten up procedures on making a charge against a property from 1994 to secure the revenue that they desperately needed. 'Social services treated those who they suspected had transferred their homes to a relative, so as to secure free residential and nursing home care, as still having those assets, and this was enforceable by law.'[54]

Unlike domiciliary care, charges for residential and nursing home care were determined by national guidelines, and these charges have played a growing part in meeting the total costs of such care, rising from around 28 per cent of the total in 1992/93 to 38 per cent in 1999/2000.[55] The main cause of this increase in charges has been the number of users who have 'failed' the means test, chiefly by having houses worth more than the minimum amount of 'assets' people are allowed to retain, as more and more people reaching old age are owner-occupiers.* Some commentators see the policy of making older people pay for residential care by selling their homes as equitable, but the 70,000 or so older people who are now forced to sell their homes to pay for their care each year not surprisingly feel angry at the way they have been treated. They feel they have contributed throughout their lives to a system that was supposed to care for them in old age, and are now being punished for having saved and become home-owners. To quote Saul Becker again:

> ... the consequence of this process [of charging] was to impoverish many elderly and disabled people. It forced them, by requiring them to spend their savings (or have their assets taken into account), from a position of independence, to a position, ultimately, of dependence on Income Support and local authority funding for the payment of their care fees. Over time, as their frailty progressed and their savings declined, they were transformed from independent citizens in the community, to financially independent users of residential care services, to the dependent poor in institutions.[56]

---

* The rates of home ownership among the sixty-five-plus age group have risen from 44 per cent in 1975 to 54 per cent in 1990. By 2001, among households containing people aged sixty-five and over, 67 per cent were owner-occupied. The actual number of older people entering residential or nursing care who owned their own homes was estimated to be around 44 per cent in 1996 (C. Hamnett, 'Housing inheritance in Britain: its scale, size and future', in A. Walker (ed.), *The New Generational Contract: Intergenerational Relations, Old Age and Welfare*, London 1996, p. 137).

NEW LABOUR AND LONG-TERM CARE

By the time Labour came to power in 1997 they were under intense pressure to redress such inequities. The main issue was the unsustainable distinction between 'health care' and 'social care'. According to one recent study, 84 per cent of care home residents need assistance with bathing and washing, while 55 per cent need help getting dressed and 45 per cent need help using the toilet.[57] But whereas any NHS patient would receive these services free of charge, for care home residents they count as 'personal care' and those with sufficient resources must pay for them. Indeed even though one in five care home residents was found to be totally dependent on care home staff, such individuals at the time of Labour's return to power were still being charged until they were too poor to pay – a process known as 'spend down', imported from the US.[58]

This highly inequitable situation could not be ignored for much longer and with a commanding parliamentary majority Labour had the opportunity to reaffirm the state's commitment to the post-1945 social contract. A Royal Commission on Long Term Care, under the chairmanship of Sir Stewart Sutherland, was asked to 'examine the short and long term options for a sustainable system of funding long-term care for elderly people ... and ... to recommend how, and in what circumstances, the cost of such care should be apportioned between public funds and individuals'.

The Royal Commission examined the evidence of actuaries, demographers, geriatricians and members of the care home industry, and also met with care home residents and their relatives. As a exercise in a policy analysis it was probably as important and as detailed as any in recent years. The report made one central recommendation: the costs of long-term care should be split between living costs, housing costs and personal care. Personal care should be available according to need, and paid for from general taxation: the rest should be subject to a co-payment by residents according to means. This, the Royal Commission, thought, was both the most equitable and the most cost-efficient policy. It concluded that:

> The most efficient way of pooling risk, giving the best value to the nation as a whole, across all generations, is through services underwritten by general

taxation, based on need rather than wealth. This will ensure that the care needs of those who, for example, suffer from Alzheimer's disease – which might be therapeutic or personal care – are recognised and met just as much as of those who suffer from cancer.[59]

Nor would this bankrupt the country: the Commission estimated that meeting the costs of 'personal care' in this way would cost between £800 million and £1.2 billion a year (at 1995 prices).[60]

By recommending that hotel and accommodation costs in care homes should be means-tested, but that personal care should be free, the Royal Commission sought to restore the comprehensive scope of free health care for all. And the Royal Commission had the backing of the public; over two-thirds believed that the state should provide free nursing and personal care as of right.[61]

Yet despite this, Labour ministers did not implement the key recommendation of the majority report. Instead it sided with two dissenters on the twelve-member commission, Joel Joffe and David Lipsey, who published a two-man minority report. For them old age was a time of 'rights and responsibilities': accordingly, the state's responsibility was only to those who were too poor to pay for all services. In their view universal benefits – provided as of right – were morally unsound, since they 'weaken the incentive for people to provide for themselves privately'. They believed that the chief responsibility for care should lie with families and other informal carers.[62] Their main recommendation, in contrast to that of the majority, was that the state should make some contribution to 'nursing care' but that 'personal care' should continue to remain a means-tested benefit.

The government published its response in an appendix to the *NHS Plan*. The government's reasoning for adopting the minority view was unprincipled and weak. The Secretary of State for Health, Alan Milburn, argued that providing free 'personal care' would only benefit those who currently had enough resources to pay for their own care, and would not fund a single additional bed for those in need. In effect he was confusing two separate issues. The Royal Commission was established to investigate who should be responsible for funding long-term care, whereas Milburn was concerned with how best to provide the much-needed additional capacity.

His reasoning not only failed to address the central issue of equity but also directly contradicted the government's stated approach to health care funding. Elsewhere in the *NHS Plan* the government had declared that charges for health care were inequitable, since 'new charges increase the proportion of funding from the unhealthy, old and poor compared with the healthy, young and wealthy. In particular, high charges risk worsening access to healthcare by the poor'.

But in response to the Royal Commission's main recommendation that charges for personal care should be abolished the government used a different argument, focusing on the most 'efficient' use of available resources. As Tony Blair told the House of Commons in February 2001, 'We have chosen not to introduce free personal care because it would cost about £1 billion, and we believe that that money would be better spent elsewhere'.[63] However neither Blair nor Milburn attempted to give an account of why abolishing charges for care in old age was not a good use of public money, nor of where these resources would be better spent. The truth was that Labour, like so many other governments before them, had simply placed older people low on their list of priorities.

The decision to continue to make long-term care a personal responsibility was greeted with outrage by those campaigning for older people. Not only had the government failed to tackle a glaring injustice but its plan to fund 'nursing' care but not personal care was, critics claimed, unworkable in practice. Drawing a line between 'nursing care' and 'personal care' would be enormously difficult and subject to arbitrary judgements by health care professionals and administrators at the local level. Indeed the use since 1995 of local eligibility criteria to determine which areas of long-term care were the responsibility of the NHS had already led to confusion and chaos. In 1999 the Court of Appeal ruled that the criteria used by some health authorities to determine who was entitled to free NHS care were unlawfully restrictive.[64] Although this led the Department of Health to issue a further clarification of NHS responsibilities, the criteria still varied from authority to authority and by 2003 significant numbers of patients in care homes were being made to pay for health services that they were legally entitled to receive free of charge. The unfairness that resulted from this confusion was brought to the attention of the Health Ombudsman, who severely criticised the

Department of Health for failing to provide 'the secure foundation needed to enable a fair and transparent system of eligibility for funding long-term care to be operated across the country', a failure that had caused 'injustice and hardship' to patients and their families.[65]

Yet it was this very system of arbitrary assessment that the Labour government now proposed to adopt as its solution to the inequities in long-term care. Under the system of 'free nursing care' introduced in April 2001, care home residents who have 'failed' the means test and are required to pay their own fees are assessed by a nurse and placed in a category according to their level of dependency. In 2003 those requiring the most nursing care received £110 a week, in the shape of an NHS contribution to their care home fees, the middle group £70, and those requiring the least care, £35.

Even aside from the arbitrary nature of the assessment process, implementing the policy has been highly problematic. The amounts paid by the NHS do not meet the actual cost of providing nursing care in care homes, and so many residents are left with a substantial amount still to pay for. Worse still, the payments are made direct to care home owners, many of whom have simply used the money to subsidise their incomes and boost their profit margins instead of reducing residents' fees. Philip Scott, the managing director of Southern Cross Healthcare Services, told the *Guardian* that Southern Cross homes were keeping the amounts paid to each resident by the NHS 'with their consent'.[66] Another for-profit provider, Westminster Health Care, proposed to cut residents' fees by only £35 whatever their assessed level of care – thus denying the more dependent residents their due entitlement.[67] Yet because the relationship between care home owners and residents is a private 'market' relationship, in which residents are merely consumers, the government has no power to intervene. Care homes cannot be prevented from increasing their fees to private patients, an action that in effect cancels out the benefits of the new payments to residents and their families.[68]

The Scottish Parliament foresaw that these difficulties would arise and in a direct challenge to Westminster, supported by all political parties in Scotland, introduced legislation in 2002 implementing the Royal Commission's recommendations. At a cost of some £125 million a year all Scottish residents over sixty-five and in need would now receive free personal care – including, but not limited to, care provided by qualified nurses. As intended by Bevan back in 1948, Scottish care home residents would be means-tested for hotel and accommodation costs, but nothing more.

The market under Labour

Labour has also encouraged the increased marketisation of long-term care, despite claiming that it had no preference for the private sector over the public sector. In April 2000 John Hutton, Alan Milburn's ministerial colleague at the Department of Health, told the House of Commons that:

> The previous government's devotion to the privatisation of care provision put dogma before the care needs of service users and threatened the fragmenta- tion of vital care services. We do not take a rigid position on whether services should be provided directly by local authorities or by the independent sector. It is the quality of care that counts.[69]

But this turned out to be only 'Third Way' rhetoric. The 'residential allowance' was phased out (thus removing the incentive for councils to place people in private care homes in order to recoup it), and the require- ment that 85 per cent of the 'Special Transition Grant' be spent in the 'independent sector' was ended. But these were token gestures which did little to worry the market because, as the long-term care market analysts Laing and Buisson noted: 'Contracting out is now sufficiently well estab- lished in local authority culture and procedures not to need protection through budgetary ring fencing'.[70] The Conservatives' policy tools had thus served their purpose. In any case the newly elected government was unwilling to jeopardise its pro-market credentials. In 1998 the then Health Minister, Paul Boateng, declared that: 'The days when a local authority could get away with an approach to residential care which was always to prefer their own provision before that of the private sector are dead and gone and will not be tolerated'. He added that if a local authority 'seeks persistently to undermine the private sector that local authority will answer for it'.[71]

So local authority provision continued to decline. Not only did the government cut the total funds from which all local authorities could borrow to invest in their own care homes from £114 million in 1994/95, to just £37 million in 1999/2000, but the legislation introduced in 1999 also made it almost impossible for local authorities to retain care homes of their own.[72] 'Best Value', a policy introduced under the 1999 Local Government Act, requires local authorities to demonstrate that their services are 'cost-effective' by comparison with those of other local providers. Given the lower rates of pay and inferior terms and conditions of staff in 'independent sector' homes, these homes will usually appear to offer 'better value'. The intention of the policy was clear. The monthly trade journal of care providers, *Community Care Market News*, commented that the 'Best Value policy … will undoubtedly mean more outsourcing of in-house residential and domiciliary care services in the future'.[73]

And so local authorities have continued to sell and privatise their care homes. According to one survey published in 2000, by 2003 local authorities in England and Wales would have sold off 137 residential and day care centres for older people at a value of some £43 million; it is a fact that the number of local authority residential care beds fell from 54,610 in 1998 to 37,310 in 2002.[74] Moreover, as a result of the pressure to achieve Best Value, for the first time ever English local authorities now purchase more domiciliary – as well as residential – care from for-profit or voluntary providers than they provide themselves, a quite astonishing turn-around considering that in 1992 local authorities provided 98 per cent of all such services. As Figure 6.2 shows, the Labour government has helped create a market in domiciliary care for older people worth some £1.4 billion in England alone.

Labour has also created a new market for independent sector providers in the form of 'intermediate care', described in Chapter 3. Officially intended to ensure that patients do not remain in hospital unnecessarily, but receive the further care they need in more appropriate settings, this new sector of care is seen as an important key to the modernisation of the NHS. Indeed the continued reduction in the number of NHS hospital beds since Labour came to power has been justified on the grounds that patients will receive 'intermediate care' instead. It is clear from government guidance that the independent sector will be the main provider of these new services, whether at home or in care homes.[75] With some 9 per cent of older patients ready and waiting to leave acute hospitals in 2002, this promises to be a lucrative new area for private provision.

Figure 6.2 The switch from local authority to independent sector provision of domiciliary care in England

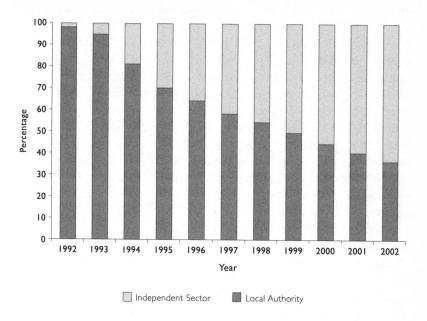

Source: Laing and Buisson, *Domiciliary Care Markets 2003*, London 2003, p. 35, Table 2.7

At the same time as it is introducing the private sector into the delivery of this new type of care, the Labour government has made intermediate care into care that can be charged for, once again blurring the distinction between NHS care and means-tested personal care provided by social services. Although it will be free for up to six weeks, it appears that patients may be liable to be billed for their non-health care needs once this period is up. The intermediate care policy thus exemplifies Labour's approach to care for older people: care for older people is increasingly something for which they can be charged, to help pay the private sector which provides it.

The state of the long-term care market in 2003

Twenty years of privatisation have left social services departments throughout the UK heavily – sometimes entirely – reliant on private operators to deliver care services for older people, and the fortunes and well-being of thousands of older people are now tied to the fluctuations of a multibillion-pound market, since the need to generate a return on investment determines how care home owners run their businesses (see Table 6.1). One consequence is the rising size of care homes. Before corporate for-profit operators entered the industry the average care home in the UK had around nineteen beds. By 2001 the average had risen to thirty. In corporate-owned *nursing* homes – as opposed to residential homes – the average number of beds is now fifty-one, compared to an average of thirty-eight for all nursing homes.[76] The larger the home the more profitable it is, since larger care home operators have access to greater revenues and are able to generate economies of scale. But from the residents' point of view larger homes may tend to detract from the quality of care and contribute to a sense of institutionalisation.[77]

Some commentators argue that private care home providers are motivated not by profit maximisation but by the needs of older people.[78] While this may be true of many smaller care home proprietors and managers, international capital views the provision of care services for older people chiefly as a source of profit. The companies that have invested in long-term care over the past decade are often venture capitalists or large conglomerates with interests in a wide range of other service sector industries. For instance Alchemy, a venture capitalist group most famous for its bid to buy the car group Rover, owns Four Seasons Healthcare, which operates over 300 care homes with some 15,000 beds.[79] Companies with hotel and leisure interests, including gambling and brewing, such as Stakis and Boddingtons, have dipped in and out of the care home market depending on the expected returns to investment in it.[80]

When care for older people becomes a profit-making industry this inevitably affects the type of care that is provided. When profit margins are tight – and the care home sector has been plagued by low levels of profitability in recent years – owners often cut back on staffing levels, freeze staff pay or cut back on 'additional' services for residents such as

Table 6.1 Top ten most profitable care home operators in the UK as of October 2003

	Number of homes	Number of beds	Revenues £m	Profit before tax £m
Craegmoor Group Ltd	313	5,828	125	28.4
BUPA Care Services Ltd	245	17,631	357	15.0
ANS Group	45	3,177	70	6.9
Care UK Plc	74	2,710	98	4.9
Barchester Healthcare Ltd	37	2,378	38	3.9
Southern Cross Healthcare Ltd	140	7,741	104	2.7
Westminster Health Care Ltd	88	5,747	142	2.5
Fourseasons Health Care Group	308	15,315	105	1.0
Runwood Homes	23	1,152	18	0.5
Life Style Care Plc	19	1,339	21	0.5

Source: Laing and Buisson, *Community Care Market News*, November 2003, p. 152

shopping trips, outings and entertainment.[81] As one voluntary organisation put it: 'Treating care homes as a financial investment means residents may be seen as a drain on resources'.[82] And when the going gets really tough, care home operators simply close their homes: since the mid-1990s, closures have led to many thousands of residents being turned out of the places that they had come to know as home. Nor are residents given much time to adjust – homes may and often do close within four weeks of the management's decision to close.[83] It is estimated that by 2003 around 74,000 care home places had been lost across all sectors since 1996, with some 800 homes closing each year from 2000 to 2003.[84] Care home owners blame the spate of closures on the low level of fees paid to them by local authorities, and there may be truth in this. But many owners have sold their homes in order to capitalise on the booming property market, particularly in the south-east of England.

While the government has funded research into care home closures 'from the provider perspective', Health Minister John Hutton told parliament that the government did not consider research into the effects of closures on residents to be 'a priority for public funding'.[85] This was certainly contrary to the view held by professionals that the 'relocation' of older people was harmful to their well-being. One consultant in old age psychiatry told the High Court in London; 'my own view is that from common experience, from my clinical experience and from an informed review of the literature, it is an inescapable truism that relocation is a stressful event and can precipitate problems of mental health, physical health and even bring forth death'.[86] Yet even the media were slow to pick up on the effects of home closure on older residents and it was only in July 2002 that the shocking story of Alice Knight, a 108-year-old woman who starved herself to death in protest at the closure of her care home in Norwich, made headline news. In most cases the true extent of the suffering experienced by many frail older people who have been 'relocated' remains unreported.

The failure of the long-term care market has had wider repercussions for the NHS as a whole. As mentioned earlier, the National Audit Office found that in 2002 nearly 9 per cent of older patients occupying NHS acute beds had been declared fit to leave hospital but had not yet done so. This amounted to more than 4,100 older patients on any given day who were deemed to be unnecessarily waiting in hospital, and one-quarter of them were found to be waiting for care home placements which were unavailable because of a lack of local capacity.[87] Aside from the distress caused to these people, the costs of market failure in this instance are transferred back to the acute hospital sector, leading to delays in treatment for other patients.

Yet rather than address the issue of market failure in the long-term care sector, the government has sought to deal with the issue of 'delayed discharge' from hospital by penalising local authority social services departments if older people remain in hospital beds longer than necessary. Under the 2003 Community Care (Delayed Discharge) Act social service departments have a minimum of two days to assess the needs of a patient and arrange a suitable package of care, or face a fine of £100 a day for every day the patient remains in hospital 'unnecessarily'. With local authorities under pressure to avoid the fine, and with long waiting lists for local care homes, many older people could be placed by social services in settings that are inappropriate for their needs or far from their families. And if an older patient or their family is unhappy with the type of care that is being proposed, social services may then inform the individual that they will need to make their own arrangements.[88] Once again the needs of older people are being sacrificed in order to make the system run more efficiently.

The failure to regulate

While the Labour government believes in the superiority of market solutions it has made some attempt to regulate the care home sector in order to protect residents from the more extreme effects of the market-place. In 1999 it announced the creation of a Commission to enforce a set of 'national minimum standards'. The National Care Standards Act of 2000 established this new regulatory framework and the National Care Standards Commission came into existence in April 2002. But Labour had not anticipated the strength of the care home lobby. Following the publication of the proposed new standards in 1999, the government came under intense pressure to water them down. The care home industry said many owners could not afford to comply with the proposed rules, and since local authorities were now almost entirely dependent on the 'independent sector' to take care of older people, the government made two crucial concessions.

The first was on staffing standards. A well-motivated, well-qualified and well-paid workforce is the key to good-quality care. But the work-force in the UK private care home sector is abysmally paid, poorly qualified and has a high turnover. One survey carried out in 2001 found that care workers in the independent care home sector were earning a maximum hourly salary of £5.05, while a survey carried out in 1996 found that two-thirds of the staff in care homes had no relevant quali-fications of any kind.[89] Indeed the workers who are responsible for caring for our most vulnerable and frail citizens are often tempted out of the caring profession to stack shelves in local supermarkets.[90] Hospital porters, cab drivers and telephonists were all found to receive similar pay to care assistants, and so it comes as no surprise to learn that around one in four care home assistants quits work in independent sector care homes every year.[91]

The urgent need for better staffing regulations in the UK's care homes became clear in 2000 when research commissioned by the charity Action on Elder Abuse found that one-quarter of all reported abuse of older people takes places in care homes, a finding that suggests that the incidence of abuse may be six times as high in such homes as in the community at large.[92] The report found that there was much less abuse where staff were properly trained and motivated. As the head of the charity pointed out: 'A member of staff who is stressed, overworked and feels undervalued is more likely to lose their temper with an elderly resident when something goes wrong'.[93] Another crucial requirement for good care is that there should be enough care workers. Evidence from the private nursing home industry in the USA shows that besides adequate pay, the ratio of carers to residents is a second key determinant of the quality of care.[94]

In 1999 the Centre for Policy on Ageing recommended that there should be one member of staff for every eight residents in a residential care home and one for every five in a nursing home, and the government initially seemed ready to adopt this recommendation.[95] But the fact that 70 to 80 per cent of the cost of running a care home consists of staff costs means that a highly trained, well-paid and substantial workforce lowers profit margins. Unsurprisingly, therefore, the care home industry vigorously resisted the imposition of minimum staffing ratios and the government backed down. Following 'consultation' it decided that the regulation of staffing levels should be determined locally and on a 'flexible' basis. Staff training standards were introduced but care homes are permitted to operate with just 50 per cent of their staff having a National Vocational Qualification. Thus old and frail care home residents were left at risk not only of poor-quality care, but also of abuse, at the hands of over-stressed and under-trained care workers.

But from the industry's perspective the government's retreat on staffing standards was nothing compared to its second crucial concession, the retreat on building specifications. In 1999 25 per cent of independent sector nursing homes had more than 20 per cent of residents in shared rooms, and 20–25 per cent of privately-run residential homes had room sizes of less than ten square metres.[96] The inadequate and inconsistent quality of the buildings that were being used to deliver institutional care thus needed addressing, and so in 2000 the government published regulations on building specifications which all homes would have to meet by 2007. A rash of home closures followed because owners, already dismayed by the low levels of fees paid by local authorities, saw the new standards as simply too onerous.

The extent of the closures began to worry the government and the issue started making headlines, with some newspapers attributing the closures not to market failure but to 'over-regulation'. At this time the government was looking to the private care home sector to provide the bulk of the new 'intermediate care' for some 270,000 mainly older people, and needed its support. So in 2002, after nearly three years of alarm and confusion, the Labour government quietly announced in the middle of the holiday season that only homes registered after April 2002 would have to meet the new specifications. The Health Secretary, Alan Milburn, had conceded on all the building standards, including room sizes, ramps, lifts, bathing facilities and single rooms. Essentially this reprieved the many substandard care homes that were already registered and saved the care home industry millions of pounds, at the expense of the conditions under which tens of thousands of older people live. Even the chief executive of the independent operators' National Care Homes Association declared that the 'extent of the concessions takes my breath away'.[97]

The power of the long-term care lobby

The closeness of the private care home industry to the inner circles of New Labour may have had something to do with the government's retreat on standards. One industry player who caught the eye of the press is the Labour Party donor and former owner of Westminster Health Care, Chai Patel, already mentioned in Chapter 1. In its 2000 survey of the most powerful people in government, the *Guardian* rated Patel the fourth most powerful individual in social care, and the eighth most powerful in health care.[98] While he owned Westminster Health Care – one of the largest private care home providers in the UK – Patel was also a member of the Cabinet Office's Better Regulation Taskforce and the Department of Health's Taskforce for Older People, and a government adviser on the elderly. He was also widely believed to have been behind the government's plans to use private care homes to provide intermediate care.[99]

Patel had voiced concerns about the government's proposed standards for the private care home industry as early as July 2000, when he warned that the plans would fail without 'greater investment' – i.e. by the government – in the sector.[100] There was something unseemly about this claim, given that Patel's own company had made a profit of £45 million the previous year and he himself was earning £433,000 a year at Westminster Health Care.[101] However his reputation as the 'fourth most powerful man in social care' went on to take a serious knock when one of his company's homes was at the centre of a widely reported scandal. Lynde House, a 72-bed nursing home in Twickenham, was accused by residents and their relatives of abusive treatment. The complaints made to the local health authority cited instances where residents had remained unbathed for months, or were left in soiled bedclothes or unchanged continence pads. Many residents had no access to call bells, and the number of staff on duty was insufficient. When three relatives raised some of these issues with the management they received letters the following day asking them to remove their loved ones from the home.[102] Nor was this a cheap, down-at-heel establishment. Some residents were paying £800 a week.[103] Yet the independent report into Lynde House found that at the heart of the home's problems were insufficient levels of staffing and inadequately trained staff – the areas that the care home lobby had successfully argued should remain regulated on a 'flexible' basis.[104] Moreover the man the government was relying on for advice on the care of older people had been in charge of the company when many of the abuses were taking place. By September 2002 Patel had stepped down from his position as government adviser when his 'tenure' with the Department of Health ended.

The care home lobby has begun to flex its muscles in other areas too. Not only have frail and vulnerable residents been the losers in the battle between the government and industry over regulation, but they are also being used as bargaining chips by the independent sector in an attempt to extract greater payments from local authorities and the government. Care home owners have been complaining for the past decade about the levels of fees paid to them by local authorities, and have attributed the large number of closures to this; and since the government has seen the privatisation of long-term care as a means of reducing the cost of care their complaint is not groundless. But with their purse strings tied by central government, local authorities have been unable to pay more. Caught in the middle have been the care home residents.

As the 'fee crisis' has worsened, the care home industry has begun to try to exploit the fact that many local authorities are now entirely dependent on the private sector and has started to mobilise its resources to fight for increased funding for the sector. English Care – and its sister organisation Scottish Care – are campaigning organisations headed by Joe Campbell, a businessman who moved into the care home sector after running security companies and commercial radio stations.[105] English Care and Scottish Care have the backing of the major corporate providers and claim to represent 80 per cent of the industry. Campbell's strategy to win extra funds was to encourage English Care members to end their contracts with local authorities unless fees are increased. 'If we are ignored', he warned the government in May 2003, 'we will have to use the weapons at our disposal and these are the beds we have'.[106] Of course Campbell was well aware that these beds contain highly vulnerable older people but he perceives correctly that it is by exploiting their vulnerability that the care home industry can win greater revenues from the government.

The strategy replicates tactics used by the US care home industry, which has a significant stake in the UK market. In one distasteful example in 2000, a care home owner in Devon threatened to evict thirteen residents just before Christmas unless the local authority increased the fees by £45 a week.[107] In 2001 members of Scottish Care refused to accept local-authority-funded residents in an attempt to enforce its demand for higher fees. Three thousand older people were left stranded in hospitals, and eventually local authorities were forced to offer care home owners an additional £27 million in order to meet Scottish Care's demands.[108] This was despite a £200 million grant from central government to enable local authorities to increase the fees paid to private sector care homes, as a result of which some local authority fee levels had risen by up to 25 per cent.[109]

There is thus a sense that the government is losing control over the care home providers on whom it now depends. Unable to prevent them from cancelling their contracts with local authorities, the Department of Health is seeking other ways to recover some control. One of the powers that is being considered by the government as a way of challenging English Care is under the 1998 Competition Act, which makes the forming of cartels in order to fix prices illegal.[110] Having unleashed market forces in the long-term care sector, the government now faces an uphill struggle to contain them.

Fighting back and seeking redress

Care home residents have not always accepted passively the treatment meted out to them by the government and the care home industry. Some have tried to fight back, to make society and the government aware that they are more than just a source of income for the industry. The High Court in London has heard numerous complaints from care home residents who have sought injunctions against home closures, and action groups have been formed to oppose care home privatisations and closures in Birmingham, Oxford, Plymouth and elsewhere. Under the title of RAGE (Residents Action Group for the Elderly) a national grassroots campaign has started to push the plight of older people in care homes higher up the local and national political agenda. As one resident in Birmingham commented, when protesting against plans to privatise her care home, 'I'm not going to sit back, we're not cattle, we're not going to be herded about. They could give us the courtesy of treating us like human beings. Just because we have complications doesn't mean our brains don't work'.[111] One care home resident, 102-year-old Rose Cottle, even made it to the doorstep of 10 Downing Street to deliver a petition protesting against the closure of her home. She was facing her second eviction in three years, as her care home in Hertfordshire was being turned over to property developers to cash in on the recent explosion in property prices.[112] But while such cases catch the media's attention and embarrass the government, they are relatively rare instances of protest from a group of people who are typically unable to agitate.

Moreover, the privatisation of residential care has adversely affected the ability of residents to seek redress against poor treatment, since their welfare is now no longer in the hands of the state but of private individuals and companies which have a right to put their own financial interests first. One example of this is legal attempts by residents to seek redress under the Human Rights Act. Initially many residents and their lawyers thought that this Act, which came into force in 2000, would provide them with a way to prevent their homes from closing, since the legislation incorporated into British law Article 8 of the European Convention on Human Rights, which creates a right to a home life. Thus when a private care home in Hampshire announced that it was to close for financial reasons, the residents sought to block the decision under the Human Rights Act, claiming that the closure would infringe Article 8. But the Act only applies to public authorities, not private individuals, unless a private body is considered by the courts to be providing a 'public function'. Despite the fact that most of the care home residents were being funded by the local authority, and that the care home was registered under the 1984 Registered Homes Act, the court ruled that the care home was not providing a public function. According to the judge the home's owner was simply a contractor to the local authority and had a right to put the company's interests first.[113] This judgement mirrors those in similar cases in the US.

So even though local authorities are now using private care homes to provide most of the care needed by older people, the latter have no recourse to the Human Rights Act against private care home owners. Residents in council-run homes can still take action against the local authority under the Act. But the number of such homes is rapidly dwindling as central government continues to force local authorities to divest themselves of their social service assets.

THE END OF SOLIDARITY?

Through a combination of rationing, charging, and means-testing the state has sloughed off more and more of its financial responsibility for long-term care, and the evolution of the system has led to wide varia-tions in the quality of institutional care, variations determined partly by geography but mainly by income. Those who have resources above the means-test level are able to pay for high-quality facilities, while those funded by their local authority are restricted to what the local authority can afford. In addition to these two tiers, if an individual qualifies for free local authority care, his or her relatives may be asked if they wish to 'top up' the basic package offered by the state. Indeed some £80 million worth of out-of-pocket payments are made by families each year to bridge the gap between what is most appropriate, or what they can afford, for their relatives, and what the state is willing to provide.[114] Thus, even where the state agrees to take on the costs of care, in fact the cost is often shared with family members who enter into a legal contract with the local authority to pay the additional amount.

And following the passing of the NHS and Social Care Act 2001 it is increasingly likely that the basic state package will be reserved for only the very poorest of older people. Under the current charging regime, care home residents are allowed to retain £12,000 worth of income or assets. Only after residents have spent their funds down to this level by paying for their care does the local authority pick up the total bill. Family members can 'top up' beyond this level, to pay for higher-quality care, but prior to the 2001 Act the resident's 'disregarded income' of £12,000 could not be used for this purpose. The care home industry, however, saw this as illogical – why should older people who were near death hold on to such resources when they could be used to pay for better-quality care? The Labour government bought this argument and since April 2001 care home residents have been allowed (at the moment in still limited circumstances) to 'top up' the fees from their own 'disregarded income', providing the care industry with what they see as 'a very important source of funding'.[115]

This much under-reported change seems to mark the completion of the conversion of the state-provided health care for frail older people into a purely residual, i.e. last-resort, service. If residents can now 'top up' from their own 'disregarded income', the basic state package may soon only be available to those who have literally no resources at all, with all others expected to 'top up' to pay for higher quality care. In effect the current two-tier system is close to becoming a multi-tier system where the state will only fully fund the wholly indigent. If this happens the idea of equal access to equal quality of care for older people will be a thing of the past. Bevan's dream of providing 'hotel-style' accommodation for all older people, irrespective of class and without stigma, will be truly dead and buried.

7

OVERCOMING OPPOSITION

When the history of the period following Labour's 1997 election triumph comes to be written people will ask with some incredulity how it was that the Labour government managed to dismantle so much of their hard-won welfare state without the public understanding what was happening, and without serious opposition from the government's own party. How was it able to convince so many people that it was still committed to comprehensive, universal and equal-access health care, when its policies were clearly running in the opposite direction?

Once again, underfunding played a key role. Because the Labour leadership had committed itself before the 1997 election to stay for two years within the spending limits proposed by the outgoing Conservatives, the NHS was subjected to a savage new financial squeeze. In many ways this reproduced the chronic underfunding of the mid-1980s under Thatcher, pushing up waiting times, leading to cancelled operations, more communication breakdowns and intensified stress. On top of this were growing strains due to the continuing process of expanding outsourcing, and the rising costs of the PFI programme, which siphoned revenues away from clinical services.

The true extent of the impending cuts in NHS services caused by the PFI was first revealed in the business cases prepared for PFI hospitals, which the incoming Labour government, in an effort to soften the blow when it adopted this Conservative policy, had made open to public inspection after the contracts were signed – a decision it no doubt regretted later. The shiny new hospital-building programme was exposed as a service reduction and hospital closure programme, and soon ran into strong opposition from the public, patients, staff, trade unions and the public watchdogs, the community health councils. The government needed a marketing strategy, and it needed ways of concealing the escalating costs and the fact that the claims of shareholders were now draining off money allocated to the NHS. There was a growing urgency to offload the political risks.

The private health care industry was also lobbying the new government. The PFI had created a new entry point to the NHS for lawyers, management consultants, the construction industry and facilities and ancillary service companies, but the health care provider industry – the for-profit hospital and insurance companies – had largely been left out in the cold. The profits to be made from privatising long-term care had been exploited by the mid-1990s, and with a government cap on funding the market was now saturated. The challenge for the private sector was to extend privatisation to clinical services. These had been relatively spared from direct privatisation except around the edges, partly because they had been protected by the system of funding but also because of the difficulty of dealing with a heavily professionalised and unionised workforce. There was pressure from the private sector abroad as well. The mainly US transnational health care corporations had identified Europe as an important new potential source of profit. They were pressing to have the scope of the General Agreement on Trade in Services extended to cover all public services, including health services, so that they could bid to take them over in any GATS signatory country.

The medical profession was also growing restless. Service cuts and loss of professional control were contributing to growing levels of stress and job dissatisfaction. Under the European working time directive, junior doctors had seen real benefits in their conditions, hours of work and remuneration. But in a situation where the workforce was not expanding, the effect of reducing junior doctors' excessive hours was to shunt work from junior to senior staff. NHS consultants who had been through the old gruelling 80–120-hours-a-week training and had been doing 'on call' for several years now found themselves doing longer hours on call, and now without the help of junior staff. GPs, too, coping with the shift of responsibility – especially for the management of chronic illness – from hospitals to themselves without adequate new resources, found their workload increasingly excessive.

Hospital support staff were feeling the impact of outsourcing and the PFI in their pay packets and terms of employment. This was especially true for staff who had been transferred under privatisation or as part of PFI contracts. Not only had their wages fallen but so too had a range of benefits. In 2000, following an acrimonious and bitter Labour Party conference, the unions were promised a review of the emerging two-tier NHS workforce that outsourcing was creating – one employed on NHS terms, and another, on much inferior terms, doing the outsourced work. A review was commissioned by the Office of Government Commerce, the body responsible for developing PPP policy for the Treasury. The review began in October 2000 but was soon abandoned, for undisclosed reasons. The *Guardian*, however, obtained a copy of the review's initial 'scoping' paper, which it said showed, to no one's surprise, that private contractors' so-called 'efficiency' savings came from cuts in staffing and some lowering of pay rates, mainly of blue-collar workers.[1]

Across the country the more militant union branches had come out on strike over these issues. In Dudley, ancillary staff went on strike for ten months in 2000–2001 against the transfer of their employment contracts from the NHS to a private consortium as part of a PFI hospital deal.[2] The consortium included SUMMIT, a large US company, in partnership with Siemens and the Bank of Scotland. The women workers involved were striking not just for themselves but for the employment rights of future employees, who would not have the same rights as transferred staff, and against the loss of beds and capacity in local health services. Although the women lost the battle, not least because there was little media support for their cause, the government seemed unnerved by these and similar actions elsewhere, and sought to find ways to accommodate some of the workers' concerns.[3]

Lastly there was the general public. The Kings Fund summarised a range of public opinion surveys which showed that 66 to 75 per cent of the public thought things had got worse rather than better under Labour.[4] There were particular concerns over Accident and Emergency departments, waiting lists and waiting times; moreover the Royal Commission on Long Term Care, discussed in Chapter 6, revealed deep public anger at the Conservatives' betrayal of the NHS promise of cradle-to-grave care.

Labour's first Secretary of State for Health, Frank Dobson, did his best to resist opening up the NHS further to the private sector, but with his resignation in 1999 the last effective defender of the NHS's original mission left the scene. Alan Milburn's appointment to replace him marked a fundamental change in pace and direction. Incremental privatisation was suddenly over. Now the government embarked on a radical acceleration in the marketisation process. New Labour's commitment to private enterprise was to be carried a large step further. The private sector was to be brought in to deliver clinical care.

But the challenge for the government was how to do this without a public relations disaster. If it was to take on the doctors, nurses and trade unions it first had to convince the public, patients and their own back-benchers that still further market-oriented changes were the solution to the problems it had inherited.

New Labour's privatising project covered the whole public sector, not just the NHS, and in conducting its ideological campaign it was able to draw on the resources of industry, the mainstream media, and a host of academics, lawyers and management consultants attracted to the power and pickings involved. Business-funded think-tanks and networks that were focused on bringing business into the public service proliferated, from the Institute of Public Policy Research, established in the 1980s, to Demos, the Social Market Foundation, REFORM, Civitas and many others. Specific to the NHS, for example, was the New Health Network chaired by Clare Perry, former chief executive at Bromley Health Authority, who had carried through a controversial PFI deal for Bromley Hospital in the face of intense and well-organised local opposition.[5] The New Health Network had 'serious business backing' from Superdrug, the discount pharmaceutical retailer, the private hospital and nursing home operator Westminster Health Care, and from KPMG, which provided launch sponsorship and staff for the New Health Network's office.[6]

The following sections show how, using all these resources, New Labour's chief tactics were to denigrate the existing public services and tout the imaginary superiority of market-based services in other countries; to add fuel to public discontent by aggravating and highlighting existing points of stress; to muzzle internal critics; to dismiss and/or contaminate scientific evidence; and, finally, to attempt to discredit, marginalise and intimidate anyone bold enough to point out what was really happening.

DENIGRATING THE ACHIEVEMENTS OF THE NHS

One of the biggest hurdles to overcome was the public's faith in the NHS. The achievements of the NHS had to be belittled, dismissed and forgotten. Supporters of universal health care were branded as sentimental and having a rosy view of the past, blind to the NHS's flaws. Politicians on all sides took to describing the NHS as a Stalinist, bureaucratic state monolith, its staff motivated by 'producer interests', not those of patients. The 'medical model' was declared part of the problem. The people now in charge of the NHS did not demur. Even the president of the Royal College of Physicians, Sir George Alberti, who later became the government's 'A&E Czar', called it 'a 1940s NHS'.[7] By 2000 the mantra that the NHS was outdated and ineffective was being repeated by the government in the preface to its White Paper, the *NHS Plan*. It declared:

> The NHS is a 1940s system operating in a 21st century world. It has:
> - a lack of national standards
> - old-fashioned demarcations between staff and barriers between services
> - a lack of clear incentives and levers to improve performance
> - over-centralisation and disempowered patients.[8]

In short, the results of fifty years of under-provision of both equipment and infrastructure, and twenty years of incremental marketisation – including the enormous political centralisation that this had required – were now blamed on the nature of the service itself.

People who had fought hard to improve the NHS found their arguments being used against it. Over the years many people had drawn attention to the NHS's weaknesses and faults, with a view to achieving its founding aims more successfully. Throughout the 1970s researchers and civil servants had striven to ensure that resource allocation did not simply reflect historic allocations and inequities. The recommendations of the government's Resource Allocation Working Party were implemented in order to improve equity in allocation of funds between areas, but sustained underfunding meant that this implied closing services in some areas to help expand them in others. Then came the internal market, which effectively swept aside equity in resource allocation. The fragmentation of the internal market and the increasing privatisation of NHS statistical data also seriously hampered the monitoring of equity in resource allocation and service use, while the abolition of community health councils, together with Labour's foundation trusts policy, reversed, in reality, the decentralisation of services and various measures that had been taken to increase local accountability. And then the NHS was denigrated as being too centralised, a postcode lottery, unresponsive to local wishes, and failing to offer 'choice'.

Eventually many media health correspondents, increasingly dependent on the drip-feed of Department of Health press releases and contacts with the government's 'special advisers', and egged on by right-wing editors, lost their objectivity. A constant media refrain became whether the NHS was 'affordable', and whether it was 'sustainable' given the challenges of an ageing population, new technology and rising patient expectations. But solid evidence on these points was hardly ever presented. Complex issues were reduced to slogans. The fact that the NHS was being deliberately shrunk was ignored, or denied.

This tendency was highlighted in 2001 when Anthony Browne, the health editor of the normally progressive *Observer*, wrote an article in which he announced that he had lost his faith in the NHS and advocated breaking it up and replacing it with a complex system of health insurance and private provision.[9] He then changed papers, becoming the environment editor of Murdoch's *Times*, and joined the Health Policy Consensus Group established by the right-wing think-tank Civitas. The Group included Dr Adrian Bull, formerly of PPP Health Care, now Carillion Health, with stakes in hospital PPPs at home and abroad; Geraint Day and Ruth Lea from the Institute of Directors; Dr David G. Green, the Chairman of Civitas, well known for his free-market views; Andrew Neil, formerly editor of Rupert Murdoch's *Sunday Times*, and now a broadcaster for the BBC; Paul Ormerod of Volterra Consulting, and author of *The Death of Economics*; and Matthew Young of the Adam Smith Institute.

Most of these institutions and individuals, having been at the forefront of the market reforms under the Conservatives, were now active in promoting a more radical privatisation under Labour.

PROMOTING THE AMERICAN WAY

Until the late 1990s the idea that any government would import the business models and techniques of the US health care system would have been greeted with incredulity and ridicule. The lack of universal health care in the USA has divided Americans culturally from their UK cousins. That the richest country in the world, with the highest spend on health care per capita, denies one in five of its citizens the basic entitlement to health care that we take for granted in the UK, is indeed hard to believe. The US health care industry's propaganda machine constantly emphasises the weaknesses of the NHS, dismissing it as a 'socialised' health care system, plagued by big waiting lists, rationing and poor-quality service.[10] But Canadians, most of whom live close to the US border and have a health care system similar to the NHS (but minus the UK's parallel private health system), invariably express their opposition to following the US model, and more and more Americans reject it too – although so far the medical insurance industry has always succeeded in thwarting state-level referendums to change it by massively outspending the reformers.

The USA epitomises all that is wrong with making health care a market matter. One-fifth of all Americans are denied access to health care because they are uninsured, and they are mainly the working poor and the unemployed. If you are insured, when you go for medical attention you must take proof of your insurance coverage – and your Visa card as back-up – since the kind of cover you have determines what kind of care, and how much, you will get. For the 300 million citizens of the USA that is the everyday reality. Nearly half of all personal bankruptcy filings are due to the costs of health care.[11] Health care cover influences all sorts of decisions people make, from moving home to changing jobs ('job-lock'). And the scale of fraud perpetrated by the private health care insurers and providers who constitute the US health care system is, as we noted in Chapter 1, breathtaking.

A colleague in San Francisco tells a story about his sister-in-law. She was thirty-five and had a brain tumour. Under the terms of her insurance policy her family arranged for her to fly from New York to San Francisco for treatment in the hospital where he himself worked. Gowned up in theatre greens, she was on the threshold of the operating theatre when her operation was dramatically stopped because the insurers claimed they had not authorised treatment. Not even the intervention of her brother-in-law, the senior physician in the hospital, or her sister, a senior radiologist, could avail. She and her distraught mother had to return home and wait for authorisation before her operation was rescheduled some months later. And if she had not had insurance she would have had to pay − if she could afford it at all.

In the film comedy *As Good As It Gets*, Jack Nicholson comes to the aid of a waitress who can't get essential health care for her child, who has asthma. She is reduced to trailing around hospital Emergency rooms because proper treatment for her child's chronic condition is not covered by her Health Maintenance Organisation or HMO. Reviewers reported that audiences all over the USA burst into spontaneous applause when she calls them 'fucking HMO bastard pieces of shit!'[12] But in spite of the well-known failings of the US system, Margaret Thatcher adopted the proposals of Alain Enthoven, a US advocate of marketised public services, to set up an 'internal market' in the NHS, while Duncan Nichol, the chief executive of the NHS who implemented the internal market, made no secret of his admiration for the USA, the market and the private sector. When he left the NHS in 1995 Nichol became Director of the Health Services Management Unit at the University of Manchester and made many visits to the USA, establishing links between US centres and the NHS management training school he ran in Manchester. In 2003 Harvard was offering courses on US health care for the benefit of NHS managers and Department of Health staff.

In 1996, when the Royal Infirmary Edinburgh approached Kaiser Permanente, a big HMO in Oakland, California, as a potential partner for the consortium putting together a bid for a PFI deal, Kaiser's medical director visited Edinburgh. On her return to the USA she said that Kaiser's conclusion was that the NHS wasn't ready for Kaiser because there were no real openings for private health care provision.[13] Little did anyone imagine that in 2003 a Labour government would ask the then chief executive of Kaiser Permanente, David Lawrence, to advise it and the NHS Modernisation Board (a body of 'experts' charged, in effect, with overseeing the marketisation of the NHS), or that it would be citing Kaiser Permanente as a model for the NHS in its key policy White Paper *Delivering the NHS Plan*.[14]

PROMOTING THE 'CONTINENTAL' SYSTEM

While the US system found favour with NHS policy-makers, efforts to sell it to the public were unsuccessful. Importing the US model had to be done by stealth. So the privatisers switched to promoting insurance systems of the kind used in continental Europe, and especially France. The French health system was now added to that country's list of attractions, along with second homes and claret. Apparently the French had found the secret of combining choice and short waiting times with a judicious mixture of for-profit and public provision — an impression that seemed to be authoritatively confirmed when in 2001 a WHO report comparing health systems put France at the top of the list.[15] It turned out that this report was an outrageously flawed piece of ideology: much of the data it purported to be based on did not exist, or had not been collected.[16] The WHO quietly dropped international comparisons. That did not stop the report being used by New Labour policy-makers to back their drive for further marketisation.

The facts about the continental health systems are more complicated. In the late 1940s most European countries looked at the emergence of the UK's new welfare state and its new health system with envy. Beveridge's five 'giants' — ignorance, idleness, disease, want and squalor — were prevalent across Europe, and in the aftermath of the war it was widely understood that Europe's reconstruction and economic revitalisation would require collective effort and collective welfare. The NHS became a role model. In the 1970s and 1980s Portugal, Spain and Greece adopted the Beveridge model of central taxation, public ownership and salaried service, preferring it to the Bismarckian systems of Germany and the Netherlands, which were universal but based on social insurance and employee–employer contributions, and the more mixed model of France.

The chief weakness of the social insurance model is that the system is organised around different employee risk pools – i.e. groups of workers in different fields, such as civil servants, groups that vary in size and in the health risks they face – and it takes complex and costly administrative arrangements to prevent cream-skimming and inequities in both funding and provision.[17] Although there is regulation – also costly – to protect the public purse, the fee-for-service system means that there are inefficiencies and inequalities in reimbursement (as well as the usual incentive to over-treat, increasing costs at the expense of patients and premiums). France, Germany and Holland were able to overcome the relative inefficiency of their systems by simply spending much more than the UK, which meant they had bigger supplies of beds, doctors and other staff (as we saw earlier in Table 3.4).

But by 2003 Germany and Holland were also dismantling their universal health care systems, cutting back on the range of benefits offered, and opening up their social insurance funds to the private insurance industry and their delivery systems to private for-profit providers. As for France, its mixed system involves very large costs, as the French public began to discover when in 2003 the government started trying to curtail the benefits offered, in order to get costs down, leading to major demonstrations and protests.[18] And the 'Beveridge system' countries – Spain, Portugal, Greece and Norway – found themselves subject to the same sort of market-driven reform as was being pushed in the UK, with a focus on finding new entry points for the private sector. Holding up the French or other continental systems as superior models had always been ideological. Now the truth was that all alike were being forced into an increasingly privatised mould.

The rate at which this happened depended to a great extent on the degree of accountability within the system, and on the power of the medical profession. In Spain and Greece, for example, the medical profession, while denigrated as 'forces of conservatism', played an important role in protecting their existing national health services from being dismantled. In the UK, by contrast, the power of doctors was diluted in the 1980s by the institution of non-clinical managers, and the BMA had long since been sidelined. Its last battle was fought over the imposition of the internal market. Attempts by the BMA to oppose the later market-based reforms were easily defeated, its members being caricatured as a greedy 'special-interest' group, resistant to change. The end of the BMA's effective independence was signalled when in 2000 it appointed as its chief executive Jeremy Strachan, a lawyer who had played a key role in the mergers of the pharmaceutical giants Glaxo and Wellcome (for which he was reported to have received a 'golden goodbye' of £1,265,000), and then again between Glaxo Wellcome and Smith Kline Beecham, to form Glaxo Smith Kline.[19] If he ever subsequently uttered a word of public support for the NHS and its founding values, it failed to receive any significant publicity.

FUELLING DISCONTENT AND AGGRAVATING STRESS: LEAGUE TABLES AND 'STAR RATINGS'

The government was walking a tightrope. On the one hand it had to be seen to be improving the NHS, on the other it needed a strategy for justifying further privatisation. The Patients' Charter introduced by John Major, which in effect defined patients as consumers, with consumer rights, had been the precursor to 'performance measurement' and 'new public management' techniques. Now hospitals were to be judged not by the care they provided but by how quickly they processed patients. The NHS adopted a factory model of care where patients were looked at like widgets on a conveyor belt, and so were constantly frustrating managers by their failure to present just the relatively standard problems that managers' 'performance targets' were premised on. For example by the 1980s and 1990s the focus was increasingly on driving down the average length of stay in hospital, in order to push more patients through the system. Staff were conditioned to think of patients as 'delayed discharges' or under other financially inconvenient labels, rather than as human beings. Under the rubric of 'payment by results', care was to be ratcheted down to the minimum, and doctors and hospitals were ranked in 'league tables' and awarded Michelin-style 'stars'.

As we saw in Chapter 4, the so-called league tables possessed no statistical validity. Few if any reputable statisticians would care to be associated with them, but there was no shortage of willing management consultants. Under contract with the Department of Health, a joint enterprise between Imperial College London and a private information consultancy firm, Dr Foster's, produces a 'Good Hospital Guide' including so-called 'league tables' of hospital performance for the *Sunday Times*. It also publishes a guide to hospital consultants, including private practice details and addresses, and a regular column for the *British Medical Journal* called Dr Foster's 'Case Notes'. In spite of having been shown to rest on statistically invalid data, Dr Foster's league tables began to be used for the overt purpose of promoting privatisation.[20] The government followed suit and produced hospital league tables of its own, despite the fact that they too contained spurious and invalid measures, and assigned Michelin-style star ratings based on them.[21] Hospitals that got no stars were said to be 'failing', and were liable to be handed over to private management – a potent threat to their managers and staff, and a humiliatingly ironic one, considering the high-profile failures of one major privatisation after another, from the Royal Armouries to Railtrack. Those hospitals that were successful and gained three stars were rewarded with new entrepreneurial freedoms, including the prospect of foundation trust status, setting them on the path to privatisation.

Just how far the league-table and star-rating culture poisoned the atmosphere in NHS hospitals, while focusing media attention on what was claimed to be evidence of the incorrigible weaknesses of the so-called unreformed public sector, will never be fully known. Doctors and nurses found themselves obliged to do whatever would improve their hospital's position in the league tables, at the expense of what their professional judgement told them they should be doing. Hospital chief executives falsified their data to improve their performance in these rankings, particularly on waiting list times, and at least two had to resign when they were found out.[22]

MUZZLING NHS STAFF

That so few doctors and nurses have spoken out against what has been done to the NHS is due above all to fear – tempered, in some cases, by financial inducements. NHS consultants are muzzled by the iniquitous system of merit awards and 'discretionary [salary] points'. Masonic-like committees meet to decide how each doctor will be rewarded. A top merit award can not only almost double a consultant's NHS salary, but also affects his or her final pension. And it is no longer other doctors but the chief executive, chairman and managers of the hospital trust who decide who receives what merit awards. Doctors need not apply unless they are willing to toe the corporate line, and little nods and whispers close to retirement age can serve all too easily to stop them blowing whistles.

Yet another weapon is clinical governance, i.e. the rules and mechanisms for ensuring good clinical practice and accountability. Much about clinical governance and audit is valuable but in the context of a politically loaded league-table culture it can have a downside: troubling or difficult doctors may find themselves subject to scrutiny and facing suspension, and then spend many months and even years struggling to clear their names.[23]

Writing in the *British Medical Journal* in 2000, the investigative journalist Judy Jones gave a disturbing account of the change in attitude towards consultant staff. For example,

> when an NHS trust in Northern Ireland reneged on promised funding for a new 10-bed drug rehabilitation unit, a consultant psychiatrist expressed his concerns to a newspaper. As a result, he was called in by his trust's chief executive who told him his actions were 'ill judged, ill advised, and detrimental to the trust'. … [Another] consultant was censured for publicly supporting a campaign to reverse a decision to close a hospital. His censure followed representations to the trust from the then minister for health in Northern Ireland, John McFall.[24]

In the past, doctors were free to speak out − in fact they were under a moral obligation to do so − if they felt it was in the interests of their patients. In a business culture, however, loyalty is said to be due above all to the shareholders. Where the survival of hospitals depends on massaging the figures and performance ratings, doctors who expose inadequacies in the system or rail against underfunding or lack of resources are seen to be criticising their own hospitals, and trusts have introduced policies requiring staff to gain the permission of their chief executives and go through the trust's press office before speaking to the press. Failure to do so has been made a disciplinary offence. Increasingly doctors are being asked to put institutional loyalty before their

professional values. Too many medical and clinical directors have told
me of veiled threats made against them when they have raised concerns
about their hospitals' policies, especially over the PFI.

POLLUTING OR DISMISSING SCIENTIFIC EVIDENCE

The strategy of polluting the science base is a well-known tactic of
industry when the evidence tells against its interests. The pharmaceutical and tobacco industries are both notorious for doing so, whether in
the use of clinical trials for marketing and promotion of their products,
or in the selective use of evidence and data in promoting their products,
or in putting scientists on the payroll who are willing to comply – and,
all too frequently, attempting to discredit scientists whose findings hurt
their bottom line. In 1998 it was discovered that tobacco companies had
paid thirteen scientists a total of $156,000 to write a handful of letters
to influential medical journals. One cancer researcher, Gio Batta Gori,
received $20,137 for writing four letters and an opinion piece to the
Lancet, the *Journal of the National Cancer Institute* and the *Wall Street
Journal*.[25] When Dr Nancy Olivieri at the University of Toronto wanted
to warn patients about the toxic side effects of a drug she was testing,
the Canadian drug manufacturer Apotex, which made the drug and was
funding the research, told her to keep quiet and threatened her with
legal action. Her hospital, which was negotiating a major donation from
Apotex, removed her from her position as director of the research unit
in her field and only reinstated her after a public outcry and protracted
legal proceedings.[26]

   As the Labour government encountered growing criticism of its
privatisation policies it began taking a leaf out of industry's book. First,
a 'rapid rebuttal unit' was established in the press office of the
Department of Health, on the lines of the one famously established in
Labour's party headquarters at Millbank before the 1997 election. The
way it worked was seen in 1999 when the editor of the *British Medical
Journal* published an editorial under the exasperated title, 'Perfidious
Financial Idiocy', to accompany a series of four papers on the PFI.[27]
The week after the editorial appeared the Prime Minister visited
Greenwich Hospital to lay the cornerstone of its new PFI building and

made a speech lambasting those he described as opposed to new investment in the NHS.[28] From then on, whenever a paper appeared that
criticised the PFI or government policy, the Department of Health
would issue a press release claiming that the analysis was wrong, or that
the researchers did not understand how care was being delivered or how
hospitals worked, but without entering into any serious exchange on
the merits of the work.

One of the four papers published by the *British Medical Journal* and
written by myself and my colleagues provided the most detailed critique
to date of PFI-funded NHS hospital projects. It attracted a robust letter
from Colin Reeves, the director of finance at the NHS Executive,
promising a response, which the *British Medical Journal* invited him to
submit.[29] Unfortunately when his response eventually came it was
judged unsuitable for publication. Reeves was invited to submit a
revised version, but this invitation was not taken up.[30] The *British
Medical Journal* eventually commissioned an investigation into why the
Department of Health had never responded to the PFI papers and
finally published the following account:

> Colin Reeves, director of finance and performance at the NHS Executive,
> promised to write an article by way of response to the *British Medical Journal*
> critiques. ... Summer, autumn, and winter passed, a new millennium dawned,
> and no article was received, nor any explanation for Reeves' evident change
> of heart. ... Rumours began to circulate of difficulties within the department
> in dredging forth suitable evidence to rebut the critics. ... Reeves did prepare
> an article for the weekly magazine the *Health Service Journal*, entitled 'Building
> the new NHS: The Private Finance Initiative'. In it he stated that 'the criti-
> cisms of the PFI have been comprehensively rebutted elsewhere'... But
> where exactly? 'We are always rebutting,' said [a] press officer later. 'We don't
> have a comprehensive record of all the articles that contain rebuttals of
> criticisms of PFI'.[31]

The government's attitude to inconvenient research data was
painfully revealed in the controversy over declining bed numbers in
acute hospitals. Declining bed numbers were the most visible indicator
of the cuts imposed by underfunding and the PFI. Within two months
of Labour's coming to power I had a meeting with Robert Osborne,

on secondment from the construction company Tarmac, who was the head of the PFI unit at the Department of Health, and Peter Coates, his number two (and later his successor). A colleague and I had asked to meet them to examine the planning base and to express our concerns over the assumptions underpinning bed numbers. To our surprise they produced a blurred photocopy of a hand-drawn graph, showing a trend line of NHS bed numbers falling steadily over the past decades. This, they claimed, justified the 30 per cent further reductions in beds that were planned in the Full Business Cases of the PFI hospital contracts that were on the point of being signed.

We responded by showing them the routine bed data in the Department of Health's statistical bulletin, which showed that the decline in acute hospital beds was levelling out, as were all the productivity gains that had helped make possible the falling bed numbers in previous years – demonstrating (what everyone in hospitals knew) that the system was under acute strain. They appeared surprised that the Department of Health collected these data, and asked for a copy. We also warned them that the bed closures occurring in the NHS long-term care sector were unsustainable and would lead to bed blockages within the hospital system. But if we thought our appeal to evidence would have any influence we were wrong. This was a political project, and the evidence would be massaged accordingly. Peter Coates continued to maintain that bed reductions played no part in PFI schemes, choosing to publish his inaccurate and misleading data in *Public Finance* rather than in the *British Medical Journal*, where NHS statisticians, doctors and public health specialists would be more likely to see them.[32]

In 1999 the Department of Health produced a similarly flawed analysis for the House of Commons Health Select Committee during the committee's enquiry into the PFI and bed reductions.[33] The Department claimed to have a report showing that no bed reductions had occurred in consequence of PFI schemes, but despite requests their paper was not published in their memorandum of evidence. We later obtained it directly from the Department of Health and found that it had measured bed closures against a baseline of the two months *following* the new hospitals' opening – whereas the bed closures associated with PFI projects naturally occur over the period, usually five years, during which the new hospital, with its reduced bed numbers, is being built.[34]

Clearly, the Department's claim made no sense, and they had good reason not to produce their evidence.

Yet another example of the government's attitude to scientific evidence followed the publication in the *British Medical Journal* in April 2003 of another article, this time showing that reductions in the bed capacity of acute specialties in the Royal Infirmary Edinburgh – reductions that had been driven by the need to make its new PFI building affordable – had led to dramatic reductions in the services delivered and numbers of patients admitted in the Lothian area compared with other areas of Scotland.[35] The article was published during the Scottish parliamentary elections in 2003, and within twenty-four hours of its appearance a press release by Dr Charles Swainson, the medical director of the Lothian University Hospitals NHS Trust, condemned it as 'completely untrue and based on inaccurate figures'.[36] In support of this accusation he cited data on inpatient and day care activity that turned out not to be statistics of actual activity but target projections from a Lothian Health Board strategy document![37]

Relying on Dr Swainson's 'authoritative' comments, however, Scotland's first minister, Jack McConnell, publicly condemned the authors' 'naïve' and 'false' arguments.[38] Then, when the false arguments were shown to be Dr Swainson's, Mr McConnell did not see fit to retract his remarks. On the assumption that the public's interest would be transient, an official silence ensued. So much for the evidence when it came to justifying the most expensive PFI hospital to date. Dr Swainson has still not corrected the public record, despite several letters pointing out his errors. However, the rising deficits in Lothian, and the high-profile media exposés of problems with the PFI contract at the new infirmar – ranging from failures of the emergency generator, so that patients had to be hand-ventilated in theatre, to the transfer of maternity cases to hospitals forty miles away caused by lack of capacity, problems with air conditioning and ventilation, and the loss of staff due to the high cost of transport and car parking – eventually forced Edinburgh City Council to launch an official inquiry in January 2004.[39] Whether the findings will attend to the planning assumptions underpinning the scheme remains to be seen.

But perhaps the most egregious example of the official attitude to scientific evidence comes from the Kaiser Permanente story. This case is especially interesting – and depressing. Instead of the government disparaging and ignoring inconvenient evidence based on sound research, in this instance (as with the WHO report mentioned on page 199) scientifically flawed evidence was not only accepted by the government even after its flaws had been exposed, but built into the policy planning process.

The story began when the *British Medical Journal*, which is considered a progressive and even radical journal by US standards, published an article by Richard Feachem, a former Dean of the London School of Hygiene, and others, purporting to show that the large Californian HMO Kaiser Permanente was cheaper and more efficient than the NHS.[40] The article was accompanied by three commentaries, including one by Alain Enthoven, the US architect of the internal market, and another by a US commentator, Don Berwick, who had been given a position on the NHS Modernisation Board, both broadly supporting the article's argument.

The response from the research community was immediate. Overnight more than seventy email responses, overwhelmingly critical of the article, poured in to the *British Medical Journal* from doctors and scientists around the world.[41] The article was found to be flawed at every level. The data had not been adjusted, as the authors claimed, for the very different populations dealt with in the two systems; inappropriate or even nonexistent data were relied on; and an elementary statistical error made complete nonsense of the overall cost comparison. Such reliable data as there were in the article actually showed that the NHS was more efficient than Kaiser.[42] Yet the article was not withdrawn or corrected by the authors or by the *British Medical Journal*, which also declined to publish an article providing detailed and quantified critique of it, on the grounds that the issues had been sufficiently ventilated in the emails available online, and that the issues were ideological not scientific.[43]

With this endorsement the Department of Health gave the green light for managers and chief executives to sign the first contracts with an American HMO, UnitedHealth Group, to provide NHS clinical services. Kaiser Permanente was cited as a model for the NHS to emulate, both in the Treasury review of the NHS funding, the Wanless Report, and in the government's 2002 White Paper, *The NHS Plan*. The head of the Department of Health's policy unit, Chris Ham, told me in December 2002 that he had teams of statisticians working on 'Kaiser 2, 3, and 4' to show just how superior to the NHS it was.

'Kaiser 2 and 3' did duly appear, compounding many of the misleading conclusions of the original article by persisting in the fallacy that meaningful policy conclusions can be drawn from the comparison in spite of the very different populations cared for by Kaiser and the NHS.[44]

This was noted by a clinical professor of medicine at the University of California, Los Angeles, who on the basis of direct experience detailed the problems with Kaiser at length before concluding: 'If one is healthy Kaiser has a relatively cheap insurance premium compared to some private insurers and delivers efficient and good care. But if one has a serious illness that is costly Kaiser leaves a lot to be desired. One cannot compare their care to that of the NHS or Medicare patients, i.e. the care extended to those aged over 65 years'.[45] But once again the damage had been done. Regardless of the evidence, the *British Medical Journal* appeared to have endorsed the 'emulate Kaiser' project. The articles were widely cited at home and abroad and became part of Department of Health thinking and propaganda. The fraudulent claims about Kaiser were taken to be true and used to promote greater privatisation of the NHS. The chief author of the original paper, Richard Feachem, some of whose co-authors had previously worked for Kaiser Permanente, was heavily engaged with the World Bank. After the paper was published he was appointed to run Bill Gates's influential Global Health Fund.

DISCREDITING AND INTIMIDATING CRITICS

The problem with attempts to dismiss or contaminate scientific evidence is that over time the evidence persists. A government can ignore it, but gradually pays a price in loss of respect and credibility. So there is a growing temptation to try to discredit and silence the source of the evidence. New Labour, committed to market policies that the evidence increasingly showed to be unjustifiable, succumbed to this temptation to an unedifying degree. Politicians eager for career advancement proved willing to use their parliamentary privilege and power to bully, threaten and intimidate, and this culture became pervasive throughout the public sector. In the field of health policy I became one of the targets. Although the account that follows is unavoidably personal, it is very much a matter of public record and is recounted here because of the light it sheds on the lengths to which Labour was willing to go to shield its market-oriented and market-driven policies from objective analysis. What happened was by no means the only attempt of its kind. The one described here, however, is particularly telling, including as it does a remarkable abuse of parliamentary privilege and of the proper functions of a parliamentary committee.

In 1997 I was asked to be a special adviser to the first House of Commons Health Select Committee inquiry into the PFI. The civil servants who were to give evidence to it had to be sent to the Civil Service College at Sunningdale for two days to be coached in the rationale for the PFI. At the end of one session, attended by the chief executive of the NHS, Alan Langlands, the head of the Department of Health's PFI unit, Peter Coates, took me aside to ask me whether it was wise or in my career interests to brief MPs against senior NHS officials. I reported the threat to Audrey Wise, an MP on the committee, and David Hinchliffe, the committee chairman, but asked that they do nothing. In retrospect I should have insisted on some action.

After Audrey Wise's tragic death from a brain tumour, and following Labour's re-election in May 2001, the government changed the composition of the committee. Its more critical members were replaced and the committee's relative impartiality disappeared. It now held an inquiry into the role of the private sector in the NHS. I was dropped as an adviser to the committee, against the chairman's recommendation, and replaced by Nick Bosanquet, a pro-market health economist, and Kingsley Manning, the director of Newchurch and Company, a pro-market health care consultancy and adviser to the government and local authorities on the PFI. In November 2001, however, I was invited to give evidence, but I was quite unprepared for the aggressive, hostile and highly ideological questions and comments I now received from some of the new Labour committee members.

The committee's report took an abnormally long time to be published, finally appearing in May 2002. About a fortnight before it was due to be published David Hinchliffe asked to see me in the House of Commons about a matter of serious concern. He told me that Julia Drown MP had tabled some paragraphs for inclusion in the report, damning my research unit and attacking me personally. She had done so against the advice of the clerks of the committee and himself. As chairman he had repeatedly asked for the paragraphs to be deleted. He had argued that such an attack on an individual witness was unprecedented and wrong, and had reminded MPs that their role was parliamentary scrutiny, not to mount assaults on individual witnesses who had none of their parliamentary privileges. He was very worried about how the unit and I would cope. He repeatedly asked me why Julia Drown was out to 'get me', and whether there was a personal element involved. As the unit's only contact with her had been through written letters questioning the basis of PFI and capital charges, there was not.

When it came to a vote most of the committee members were absent and the offending paragraphs were voted in by 3 votes to 2. All the chairman could do now was give me advance warning to be prepared for a destructive and vicious attack that he said he would do his best to defend me against. He said he realised the attack would have a serious impact in the short term, although he felt personally that all our work would be vindicated. The report was duly published, including the following misleading assertions about our evidence:

67. Furthermore, the HPHSRU's [Health Policy and Health Services Research Unit] assertion that it was never a good thing in the NHS to have increased capital charges funded by a revenue budget, for example by staff savings, was dubious. Many projects in the NHS, such as MRI scanners and ward reconfigurations, fall into this category and have led to better patient services. This has raised serious questions about the HPHSRU's ability to analyse rationally the finances of the NHS. An MRI scanner, by scanning patients more quickly, could allow patients to have a better service whilst reducing the need for radiographer time, which could at least in part, pay for the additional capital costs.[46]

However no such assertion had been made. The exchange which took place was actually as follows:

Q. [Julia Drown] Do you accept the point that sometimes in the NHS it is good to spend more on capital and less on medical staff because it gets a better service?

[Professor Pollock] I accept the point but not from the revenue budget. When you do it from a cash restrained, under-resourced revenue budget, you should not be using that for your capital. You should have proper capital flows and a proper system of capital funding.[47]

The point at issue was deliberately obfuscated in the paragraph Drown got inserted in the committee's report. The point was not whether capital spending can lead to 'better patient sevices' – of course it can. The point was whether capital investments should be paid for out of the revenue budget – i.e., out of the flow of funds available for current spending. If an investment leads to a reduction in current spending by more than the cost of the investment – e.g. by saving on staff – then it may be justified to finance it out of the revenue budget from which staff salaries are paid. But if it costs more than any such savings, and if the revenue budget is capped and already underfunded, it will mean a reduction in services overall, not an improvement. This was the point I had made, as Drown surely understood. She chose to twist a statement about funding into an argument against any switch from labour to capital, or from medical staff to MRI scanners.

The report went on to accuse the unit of a 'lack of sound analysis' and 'antagonistic extreme views', without offering any evidence of either. The aim seemed to be to use the protection of parliamentary privilege to try to discredit researchers whose findings failed to endorse government policies. The report was also a gift to the private sector because of its endorsement of the PFI. By now the policy of the PFI and PPPs was not just public sector policy, but a growing UK export. But as PPP was spreading globally, so too was the resistance from trade unions, academics and local people everywhere. The work of the unit had an international profile and we were deluged with invitations to go to Canada, the US, Australia, South Africa and various countries in Europe to help provide an analysis of PPPs. The effect of these inter-ventions was not just national but international. The growing opposition to the policy in these countries was significantly reliant on our work. From the government's point of view we had to be deni-grated, and preferably silenced.

It was hard for us to limit the damage done by Drown's attack. Our resources were very slim, lacking as we did the funding offered to the promoters of PFI/PPP by the private sector. We published a rebuttal, and the *Guardian* and *Private Eye* examined Drown's questionable motives.[48] Roy Hattersley also intervened. As the Health Select Committee report was going to press a launch meeting was held for the think-tank Catalyst, with Roy Hattersley as chair. I took the opportunity to tell him what had happened and he obviously took other soundings and then wrote a magnificent article in our defence, as did a number of senior academics from across the world.[49] The chairman of the Health Select Committee and a number of MPs also made supportive speeches in parliament.[50] But the pressure on the unit was destabilising and time-consuming. Much of our work had to be put on hold while the unit fought for survival. This, no doubt, was the object of the attack.

8

THE EMERGING HEALTH CARE MARKET

The NHS is being dismantled and privatised. Very soon every part of it will have been 'unbundled' and commodified. It began with ancillary services such as cleaning, catering, laundry and portering. This was rapidly followed by finance, buildings, maintenance and repairs, creating a £1 billion market on which the fortunes of giant corporations rest. Now the same process is being extended to core support services like diagnostics, information technology, equipment procurement and maintenance, and management. Market forecasters estimate a £10 billion market over the next five years in NHS information technology alone.[1] Finally clinical services themselves are being broken up. Private health care companies now provide routine elective diagnostic and surgical interventions, primary care services, screening, prevention, intermediate care and long-term care. And what remains of the NHS is itself being floated off as a series of small businesses in the shape of the 'foundation' hospital trusts, whose priorities will be financial.

Also deeply involved are the Big Four companies of auditors and management consultants, and the corporate law firms responsible for drawing up hundreds of thousands of contracts and subcontracts with all these private providers. Legal contracts now govern the running and operations of all PFI hospital buildings and their management, as ownership is transferred to the private sector, and in the same way the supply of clinical services will in future be determined not by strategic planning bodies but by the market through contracts with suppliers.

Increasingly every aspect of health care will be provided under a complex web of contracts which will be difficult if not impossible to monitor and enforce – contracts that bind the government and the public for at least twenty-five years, with seemingly little hope of ever regaining control. The high-profile private sector failures of the railways, government information technology systems, the Benefits Office, the Passport Office, the Channel Tunnel and long-term care all illustrate the difficulties governments will face when confronted by the monopoly power of private suppliers of health services. On top of this the Labour government is actively contemplating the imposition of user charges for service 'upgrades', including the so-called hotel costs of hospital patients, spelling the final end of health care as an equal and universal right.[2] The disaster that is unfolding is overwhelming in its complexity and its magnitude. Even rail privatisation looks modest alongside it.

THE NEW BUSINESS MODEL AND WHAT IT MEANS

It is easy to lose sight of the benefits the NHS secured: integrated hospital services with minimal internal administrative costs; district general hospitals, bringing specialist services for all but the rarest conditions within reach of every family; the evolution of general practice to offer 24-hour primary care by doctors trained for the job, and continuity of care for everyone; robust structures for data collection and planning in order to match resources to needs; the education and training of medical staff; and the gradual equalisation of service provision across the country, while still allowing for experimentation and innovation that have made British clinical practice and research among the best in the world.

Today the institutions that made the NHS strong, economical and popular are being dissolved and overturned. In their place are market mechanisms: invoicing, customers, segmented risk pools, legal contracts, and a myriad of competing suppliers. The NHS's institutional memory – the memory of an alternative way of organising health care – is being rapidly eroded. Civil servants in the Department of Health and the Treasury, and hospital chief executives and board members, now accept only one model of the way services should be delivered: the business model. The public service paradigm is denigrated and ignored. Margaret Thatcher's adviser, Sainsbury's Roy Griffiths, gave us the supermarket model of care, while Gordon Brown's adviser, NatWest's Derek Wanless, gives us corporate mergers and public–private partnerships. A new business dynamic is taking charge of the ways in which services are provided and patients are responded to. The dramatic costs involved – in terms of the loss of equal access and universal standards, as well as of money – are concealed by claims of 'commercial confidentiality' and by tearing up the once-exemplary systems of NHS accounting.

But large institutions are hard to destroy when they command public trust. New Labour's 'reformers' have had to fall back on the rhetoric of business, portraying the NHS as a failing state monolith, a dinosaur whose time is past. How many times have we all listened to conversations in which one side goes like this: 'The NHS is a multibillion pound business. With over a million employees it's the second largest employer after the Red Army. No one can run a business that size. No wonder it's bureaucratic and inefficient. The people I meet don't care whether it's BUPA or Boots providing the service so long as the government is paying for it. What matters is quality. In any case, with an ageing population and the ever-rising costs of new technology, we can no longer afford the NHS. The demand for health care is infinite, so rationing is inevitable. Why shouldn't those who can afford to, pay for some extras, and free up resources for those who can't? Why should those who want to not go privately or pay for their own care? Public expectations are so much higher. What people want today is choice.'

Masquerading as rational arguments, these soundbites permeate public discourse. Like prions, vicious sequences of malevolent proteins, they replicate in the media and insert themselves in the brains of policymakers, and eventually lethally infect government White Papers and legislation. Honest and transparent health policy-making would require close forensic scrutiny of all the NHS's activities: its planning, its provision, its costs, its income, its expenditure and its outcomes; above all, of how its core principles and functions are embodied in practice. It would require much of the kind of analysis we have attempted to give in various parts of this book. But the job of the political spin-doctors is not analysis but the propagation of market prescriptions. These have already been applied across the rest of the public policy spectrum. Now it is the turn of patients. Instead of a democratically accountable health service we are to be customers of health businesses, ultimately interested in us only for our contribution to their bottom line.

Of course accountability takes many forms, but in the case of health care what most of us broadly understand by it are the institutions required for proper governance. These include robust financial reporting systems, transparent mechanisms for ensuring equity of resources, planning processes capable of responding to population needs for service, monitoring systems capable of determining when things have failed or are inadequate, and a variety of mechanisms to ensure the views and needs of patients, staff, carers, relatives and the public are heard and responded to. All of these depend on having good data and planning systems in place. None of them exists in the fragmented 'mixed economy' health care market to which the NHS is being reduced.

One consequence of the market is that it is now virtually impossible to track NHS expenditure. Take, for example, management costs, which include the costs of invoicing, communications, information technology, human resources and numerous other services. Under the internal market NHS bodies were required to keep management costs below 7 per cent of total income and the Department of Health undertook to ensure that this happened. But NHS Trusts were able to conceal and massage their management costs by excluding contracted-out services, or by allocating management staff to different personnel categories. Now, although every hospital has a public relations and communications office, no data are available, in aggregate or for individual hospitals, on how much is being spent on employing staff directly or on contracted-out services.

And the lack of transparency is set to worsen. Recognising the huge new costs of administering and implementing the market with its pricing system and contracts, in 2004 the government lifted the ceiling on management costs. Moreover the move away from standard definitions and systematic data collection will make it increasingly hard to tell how new resources allocated to the NHS are being spent. An alphabet soup of definitions and standards is emerging which means that it will be difficult if not impossible to quantify the distribution and supply of resources, including beds and staff, in relation to the size of the local population and its health needs, or to measure inequities in provision. John Reid, the Secretary of State for Health, has notoriously said, 'wherever possible I want to stop collecting data'.[3] There are also increasing barriers to accessing information. Some NHS trusts now charge members of the public (their real shareholders) for a copy of their accounts – something no private company would dare to do to its shareholders.

THE POWER OF MARKET INCENTIVES

Above all we need to understand what the new structure of incentives in the system as a whole will make it do. The new financial system that is currently being put in place is based on market incentives. Resources are no longer distributed in line with aggregate measures of the health needs of every locality and population mix. In the new business-oriented regime, 'money will follow patients' and hospitals will be paid by 'results'. In theory, patients will go where the services they want are on offer, and the government will pick up the bill on the basis of the price list in the 'national tariff'. But the reality is bound to be different, because foundation trusts are being established as businesses, and so will have to perform like businesses. The new regulator, Bill Moyes, sees the process of establishing foundation trusts as 'equivalent to floating a company on the stock market'. They must have secure cash flows from their contracts with primary care trusts and sound business plans, and behave accordingly.

This means that the main focus of chief executives and trust boards is now unavoidably on strategic developments that will enhance their cash flow, not least mergers and takeovers. Weaker hospitals will be absorbed, and, as in the US, residents in some areas will find that their local hospital services, including Accident and Emergency departments, come to be closed, and their assets liquidated – as they already have been, in many places, as a result of the internal market and the PFI hospital-building programme. Futhermore, the national tariff creates an incentive for hospitals to cherry-pick lucrative treatments, specialties and doctors, and avoid those that involve higher risks and low returns

— notably emergency and intensive care, and the treatment of chronic illnesses. Staff and resources will gravitate towards fashionable treatments and specialties.

The government pretends that the national tariff or price system now being introduced is a fair system. But the facts indicate otherwise. Not only does the cost base of hospitals vary according to inherited differences in their plant and the local need for hospital services, but the way in which the government can change the book value of trusts' assets, and/or inject subsidies, makes the system arbitrary. Chief executives of would-be foundation trusts have been negotiating with the government over the size of their 'dowries' and cash flows. Those first off the block will get their land and assets valued at knock-down prices, keeping their apparent costs low. In addition the government is making extra capital available to them and allowing them to borrow capital from the NHS Bank at low rates of interest. Chief executives are also negotiating over the pricing system itself, so that it will serve their needs best. Like fund-holding and the PFI, foundation trusts are a political project and cannot be seen to fail. But their success will be achieved at the expense of health care for all.

The new structure of incentives will affect the outlook of the NHS workforce. As one bemused public health consultant remarked on joining one of the new primary care trusts: 'Nowadays anything seems to go — there don't seem to be any professional barriers to farming out work to anyone, regardless of their qualifications'. Anyone who has been a hospital patient knows and appreciates the difference between the regular nursing staff, however overworked they are, and the agency staff who tend to cover on nights and who may be perfectly competent but don't know the patients and won't be responsible for you tomorrow. Eventually this detached, contract-limited attitude will become the norm for all NHS staff, if trusts' overriding financial goals are to be met.

Performance targets will increasingly focus on the bottom line. Under the new GP contract, for example, payments are linked to performance measures such as the percentage of patients whose blood pressure is maintained within strictly defined limits. GPs are already concerned that there will be a temptation to manipulate the readings in borderline cases, and to treat even mild blood pressure problems with drugs for quick results, rather than treating the disease in a holistic way, i.e. focusing on diet, exercise, stress and lifestyle. The new contract also focuses on 'disease management' for diseases where the easiest thera-peutic remedy is drug intervention. The new performance measures are largely linked to pharmaceutical interventions of one sort or another, and the pharmaceutical companies have been swift to respond, using strategies developed in the US.

GPs may find it is not worth their while to provide some services for which they receive no specific reimbursement. For example they will now be paid for achieving specific percentages of patients who have received flu vaccinations or childhood immunisations by a specified date in the year. Once that date is passed, although dedicated GPs will continue to try to reach patients who have still to be immunised there will be no further financial incentive to do so. Core public health func-tions are thus put at risk.

And forget 'diversity' and 'choice'. Physical access is already being curtailed by the closure of local hospitals and the movement of services to out-of-town locations, involving higher transport costs. The gate-keeping role of GPs is being replaced by numerous other gatekeepers such as NHS Direct and private 'out of hours' services. Each change has the effect of placing new barriers to integration and continuity of care. Some patients – mainly elderly people facing discharge from hospital, but still in need of 'intermediate' care – are now being 'triaged' (i.e. sorted into an order of priority for treatment) on the basis of their ability to pay (or their eligibility for financial support), not on the basis of their need for care. And once people have become used to this it is easy to envisage that ability to make 'co-payments' – i.e. pay fees – for various aspects of hospital care could become a criterion of selection too.

The new system of risk assessment, under which providers will be reimbursed according to the complexity of the conditions they treat, could generate several thousand different Diagnosis Related Groups (see pages 120–21). Each of the millions of NHS patients treated annually will need to be categorised, coded and then billed and invoiced for. In the USA this results in fraud to the value of billions of dollars of tax revenues annually. New Labour make much of the fact that this system is now also being used across Europe, but neglect to mention that its origins lie the private medical insurance industry of the USA, and that its current adoption in Europe reflects the way in which the other European health services are also being broken up and privatised. In the US, the transaction costs involved in billing and marketing can account for 30 per cent of every dollar spent on health care, and Britain is set to follow suit.[4]

The new financial system creates conflicts between the interests of patients and the interests of the hospitals. The US experience shows that the reimbursement of hospitals according to risk inevitably results in two kinds of adverse behaviour. First, hospitals claim more than they should by exaggerating patients' needs and the kinds or amounts of treatment they have been given; and second, hospitals select patients in order to avoid taking on those with complex problems. Ways are found to discourage the admission of patients with conditions calling for treatments that do not generate surpluses.

At one heart hospital in Phoenix, Arizona, the head of the service was overheard saying to his junior staff: 'Every patient in this hospital needs an operation, it's your job to find out which one'. The surgeon, who also owned the hospital, had a weekly radio programme on which he advertised his services, recruiting patients from among the 'snow birds' – mainly wealthy retirees from northern states who arrive in droves every winter. The UK's new performance measurement system – which requires hospital trusts to break even, and league tables that will continue to rank hospitals and doctors – will have similar effects. Among other things, the patient's advocate role of doctors and nurses will become much weaker. Nothing must be done that jeopardises the bottom line.

In other words, the new incentive system has nothing to do with need and everything to do with the supermarket model of care. 'Payment by results' always means over-diagnosis and over-treatment of some, and neglect and under-treatment of others.

'MEMBERS'

The switch to having a limited number of 'members' of hospital foundation trusts drawn from local residents, patients and hospital staff, in place of the notion that hospitals belong to all of us (see Chapter 3), is a central and so far neglected plank of the marketisation project.

Membership is the soulmate of the market, eroding the concept of universal rights and automatic entitlement and allowing an appointed elite of chief executives and directors to decide, in effect, who belongs and who doesn't.

Foundation trust 'membership' is touted as a democratic innovation. But the first wave of trusts applying for foundation status have minute membership bases: a few hundred self-selected individuals out of hundreds of thousands of local residents. And the power granted to members in foundation trust constitutions, like the power of individual small shareholders in the private companies that foundation trusts resemble, is intended to be negligible. What foundation hospital trusts actually stand to gain by having members – among whom patients seem likely to predominate, since they become members automatically – is a potential market for health insurance policies, and a means for 'market-testing' user charges or co-payments – as some chief executives are already recognising. And in spite of Secretary of State John Reid's denials, co-payments are very much on the agenda that is being developed in Downing Street for a third New Labour term of office. They are also close to the hearts of the Conservatives, who in addition are committed to moving to health insurance in place of tax funding. In general, the Conservative Party, with its talk of 'patient passports' – in effect, vouchers – is signalling that it will pick up where Labour leaves off. Labour's focus has been on privatising the delivery of health care, while the Conservatives are focusing on privatising *funding*, through private insurance and co-payments. The Conservatives' promise to see spending on the NHS increase even more than under New Labour reflects this intention, combined with their appreciation that New Labour's 'mixed economy of health care' will need hardly any adjustment to become the means of funnelling still more tax revenues and 'co-payments' to the private health care industry.

FROM RATIONAL PLANNING TO A MARKET 'REGULATOR'

The systems created under the NHS for planning universal health care have been dismantled. An early casualty has been public health. The disastrous consequences of dispensing with public health measures that protected animal husbandry and the food chain were all too evident in the government's responses to the foot-and-mouth and BSE epidemics. In each case, commercial and trade imperatives overrode public health precautions. These processes are now at work within the NHS. Over £3 billion is being spent on information hardware for the NHS, but the data sets that are required to support the rational planning and evaluation of services are being neglected and even dismantled. For example the long-awaited 'community data set', which would have provided data on patient needs and the distribution and supply of services such as chiropody, physiotherapy and speech therapy, has been abandoned.

With increasing fragmentation among competing providers and a diminution in the requirements laid on them to provide data it is becoming increasingly hard to see how any rational oversight can take place. Anyone trying to study population planning for health services in the USA soon discovers that the concept of rationally planned service provision is entirely unfamiliar to health policy-makers there. The only system they know and understand is the market, which is also the standard against which visiting US policy advisers to the Department of Health now judge our success. Many US doctors cannot think outside the HMO model, according to which quality equates with financial performance and incentives, and increasingly this is the gospel we are being taught.

In the market, effective power will reside with the boards of directors of hospital trusts — most if not all of which will eventually be foundation trusts — plus the larger private companies providing NHS services, supervised by the independent regulator. The government argues that this structure will return services to local control, but a glance at foundation trusts' constitutions and the experience of the first wave of trusts to apply for foundation status shows this to be a myth. Out of more than 2 million people served by the first ten such hospitals, only 34,000 residents and patients registered as 'members', and including hospital staff only 20,000 people actually voted in the elections for the 'governors' to whom the directors are nominally responsible.[5] The new NHS will be accountable only to a regulator with extraordinary power but very limited health responsibilities. His duty is to issue the licences to foundation trusts and to determine the range of services they can provide. The prices of the trusts' services, however – the national tariff – will continue to be set by the Department of Health, while quality, safety and performance will be monitored by the many advisers who will in turn be accountable to the regulator. It is not hard to see that in the absence of a strong statutory requirement to ensure universal access and equity, and without mechanisms to do so, the regulator's function will be above all to make the market work, and this will always prevail. The legislation imposes almost no restrictions on what the regulator can and cannot do. Faced with a choice between liquidating a hospital trust that is in danger of bankruptcy, or closing a major service, he is bound to agree to at least a partial service closure, or the imposition of some new charges, or both.

All this is defended in the name of giving people 'choice', when the opposite is really occurring. When people are really sick they are seldom in a position to exercise rational choice, as Tony Blair found when he had a heart problem – doctors alone were in a position to decide where the best care was to be had, and he got it. Most people don't know what health care they need, or, if they have to pay for it, whether they can afford it; nor can they pick and mix according to what happens to be on offer that week. The supermarket model of health care implied in politicians' rhetoric is a sham. Before long people will get a kind of choice that they can make: to take out insurance – and be prepared to find the 'co-payments' (i.e. fees) and the 'deductible' (excess) – or go without.

THE REAL CHOICE

The NHS was not an experiment, nor was it a mythical utopia. For more than fifty years it has delivered high-quality care on the basis of need to most patients most of time. Although its highest aspirations have not always been fully achieved, its success inspired many other countries to follow suit, with similar success. Now it has been made into a laboratory for market-based policy prescriptions. Across Europe and much of the rest of the world, countries are dismantling their universal health care systems. The regulations that once protected public ownership and control are being rewritten in favour of private sector interests.

Most attention has been paid to the role of the WTO and international financial institutions such as the IMF and the World Bank. But the trading blocs that make up the WTO are translating the WTO rules into domestic law so that they will have domestic force. National states will no longer retain sovereignty over social welfare issues. As with agriculture and food policy, draft directives currently before the EU are extending its reach to health and social care, redefining them as economic services subject to the terms of trade treaties and competition policy. Trade bodies and tribunals rather than democratic institutions responsible for education and health will increasingly determine their future.

What is at stake is whether we want to break up one of the key bonds that make our society more fair, more civil and more gentle than that of the USA. The NHS was an effort to remove health care, and so the risk of ill-health, from both the political and the market arena, to make the right to health as equal as the right to vote. What is happening is the destruction of that. The social and political consequences will be more far-reaching than those involved realise.

What is to be done, with so little time available before the Dr Jekyll of Britain's National Health Service becomes the Mr Hyde of the US health care industry? First, the structures that make possible planning and a population focus need to be restored and then strengthened, to make their democratic accountability more immediate and far-reaching. Services need to be made accountable to local people directly, not through shadowy pseudo-democratic boards that meet only three times a year. Second, the enormous transaction costs and waste associated with the market need to be exposed and brought to an end. This means opening up the market's transactions to scrutiny, showing how corporate shareholders are making extraordinary claims on scarce public resources, and how much of the new money promised for the NHS disappears in private sector duplication, transaction costs and fraud.

It is not hard to see that if the NHS had been funded since its inception on the scale of other EU health systems, the public discontent that the privatisers were able to exploit could have been averted. Now the benefits of improved funding – to the extent that they are not soaked up by hospital trusts' accumulated deficits, or siphoned off into private sector profits – will be attributed to the very market 'reforms' that underfunding allowed successive governments to introduce.

Future governments will say that it was the NHS that failed, and this will become harder and harder to dispute because it will be increasingly difficult, if not impossible, to show where the money went. This book is an attempt to show that the NHS has not failed and need not fail. What is required now is not reform but revolution – a quiet, collective and reflective revolution of the sort that brought the NHS into being in the first place.

NOTES

1 MARKET PRESCRIPTIONS

1 To take one example among many, when in May 2004 Nestor Healthcare, an employment agency, misjudged the size of the new market for providing 'out of hours' GP services, its share value dropped 36.5 per cent and its chief executive resigned (*Guardian*, 4 May 2004).

2 Paul Foot, 'Medes and Persians', *London Review of Books*, 2 November 2000.

3 Andrew Smith MP, *Hansard*, 31 October 2000, Column 339W; Department of Health, *Sold on Health: modernising procurement operation and disposal of the NHS estate*, London 2000.

4 Derek Wanless, *Securing Our Future Health: taking a long-term view,* Final Report, HM Treasury, London 2002.

5 Kevin Maguire, 'Union attacks Milburn election role', *Guardian*, 8 May 2004; and http://www.bridgepoint-capital.com.

6 Luke David, 'Bart's private bidders enjoy unhealthy ties', *Highbury and Islington Express*, 25 October 2002.

7 www.hcp.co.uk.

8 David Batty, 'Chai Patel, Westminster Health Care', *Guardian*, 25 September 2002.

9 www.prioryhealthcare.co.uk.

10 Tash Shifrin, 'Retail chief takes foundation reins', *Guardian*, 4 December 2003.

11 'Drug adviser quits over policy switch,' BBC News, 10 July 2002,

www.news.bbc.co.uk.

12   *Private Eye*, No. 1087, 22 August–4 September 2003, p. 6.

13   Adele Shevel, 'Healthcare groups in UK bids', *Sunday Times* (South Africa), 27 July 2003.

14   John Carvel, 'Controversy at the cutting edge', *Guardian*, 3 December 2003.

15   'Netcare signs big UK health services deal', *Business Day*, 25 September 2003.

16   'Foreign eye ops under scrutiny', BBC News, 23 September 2003, www.news.bbc.co.uk.

17   www.healthmarkpartners.com.

18   Howard Berliner, 'American Booty', *Health Service Journal*, 6 July 2000.

19   For details of all these cases and other instances of health care fraud in the US, see the US Department of Justice website: www.usdoj.gov.

20   The Quorum Health Group, the USA's largest hospital management company, which was also involved in defrauding the US government, paid back $85 million in April 2001. According to the Health Policy Network, the FBI estimated that in the years 1990 to 1995 health care fraud in the USA totalled no less than $418 billion (*Health Care – Private Corporations or Public Service? The Americanisation of the NHS*, Third Report of the Health Policy Network, London 1996, pp. 29–32.)

21   Anthony Barnett and Solomon Hughes, 'UK's elderly care plan run by US "cheats"', *Observer*, 10 November 2002. The data in the following two paragraphs are taken from the same article.

22   Robert L. Kane, Shannon Flood, Gail Keckhafer *et al.*, 'Nursing home residents covered by Medicare Contracts: early findings from the EverCare Evaluation Project', *Journal of the American Geriatrics Society*, Vol. 50, April 2002, pp. 719–29; for United HealthCare's support for Bush and Cheney see www.whitehouseforsale.org, and United HealthCare's 2003 Annual Report.

23   Barnett and Hughes, 'UK's elderly care plan run by US "cheats"'.

2   THE REAL COST OF MARKET PRESCRIPTIONS

1   David Price, 'Lessons for health care rationing from the case of Child B', *British Medical Journal*, Vol. 312, 1996, pp. 167–9.

2   Barbara Millar, 'Short of patients and full of anger', *Health Service Journal*,

13 August 1992, p. 11.

3 The increase in prescription charges throughout the 1980s and 1990s meant that the cost of medicines increased particularly for those who suffered from many chronic diseases such as asthma, hypertension and arthritis, and who were not exempt from prescription charges due to their income. GPs began issuing private prescriptions to patients whenever the cost of medicines was less than the prescription charge. This also had advantages for GPs since it reduced the pressure on their prescribing budgets. See Iona Heath, 'The creeping privatisation of NHS prescribing', *British Medical Journal*, Vol. 309, 1994, pp. 623–4.

4 Sanjiv Sanchev, *Contracting Culture: from CCT to PPPs*, UNISON, London, November 2000; UNISON/East London Community Organisation, *Pay and Conditions claim for Private Contract Staff – East London Health Trusts*, UNISON, London, 5 July 2002; Auditor General for Scotland, *Hospital Cleaning*, Audit Scotland, Edinburgh, January 2003.

5 Joint Working Party of the British Medical Association, Royal College of Surgeons, Royal College of Physicians, 'Provision of general acute hospital services', London 1998; Royal College of Physicians, 'Future patterns of care by general and specialist physicians', London 1996.

6 Department of Health, 'Keeping the NHS local – a new direction of travel', London 2003.

7 Harriet Harman MP, *Hansard*, 12 March 1996, Column 821.

8 House of Commons Health Committee, 'Public Expenditure on Health and Personal Social Services 1999', HC629, London, June 1999, Table 4.8h; Sean Boyle and Anthony Harrison, 'PFI in health: the story so far', in Gavin Kelly and Peter Robinson (eds), *A Healthy Partnership – the future of public private partnerships in the health service*, Institute of Public Policy Research, London 2000.

9 Declan Gaffney, Allyson M. Pollock, David Price and Jean Shaoul, 'PFI in the NHS – is there an economic case?', *British Medical Journal*, Vol. 319, 1999, pp. 116–19.

10 Allyson Pollock, David Price and Matthew Dunnigan, 'Deficits before patients: a report on the Worcester Royal Infirmary PFI and Worcestershire hospitals reconfiguration', UCL, London 2000, p. 5.

11 Allyson M. Pollock, Jean Shaoul and Neil Vickers, 'Private Finance and "value for money" in NHS hospitals: a policy in search of a rationale?' *British Medical Journal*, Vol. 324, 2002, pp. 1205–9.

12 Allyson M. Pollock, Matthew G. Dunnigan, Declan Gaffney, David Price and Jean Shaoul, 'Planning the "new" NHS: downsizing for the 21st Century', *British Medical Journal*, Vol. 319, 1999, pp. 179–84.

13 Colin Leys, 'Intellectual mercenaries and the public interest: management consultants and the NHS', *Policy and Politics*, Vol. 27, No. 4, 1999, pp. 447–65.

14 K. Janzon, S. Law, C. Watts, A. M. Pollock, 'Lost and confused', *Health Service Journal*, 9 November 2000, pp. 26–9.

15 House of Commons Health Select Committee, 'Public Expenditure on Health and Personal Social Services 2001', HC242, London 2001, Table 5.6.1.

16 HMSO: Statutory Instrument 2003 No. 1196 The Community Care (Delayed Discharges etc.) Act (Qualifying Services) (England) Regulations 2003.

17 Department of Health, 'Proposed amendments to the National Health Service (Charges to Overseas Visitors) Regulations 1989: A Consultation: Summary of Outcome', December 2003.

18 John Carvel, 'Foreigners will be vetted to get NHS treatment', *Guardian*, 31 December 2003.

19 John Carvel, 'Claim on cost derived from debt agency', *Guardian*, 31 December 2003.

3   PRIVATISING THE NHS: AN OVERVIEW

1 See e.g. David Osborne and Ted Gaebler, *Reinventing Government: how the entrepreneurial spirit is transforming the public sector*, Plume, New York 1993.

2 Charles Webster, *The Health Services Since the War*, Vol. I, HMSO, London 1988, pp. 137 ff.

3 John Mohan, *A National Health Service? The Restructuring of the Health Service in Britain since 1979*, St Martin's Press, New York 1995, pp. 13–15.

4 *Report of the NHS Management Inquiry* (the Griffiths Report), October 1983, pp. 12 and 14.

5 Charles Webster, *The NHS: a political history*, OUP, Oxford, 2nd edition, 2002, p. 203.

6 Office of Health Economics, *Compendium of Health Statistics 2003–2004*, London 2003, Table 3.3.

7 Jane Wills, *Mapping Low Pay in East London*, a report written for TELCO's Living Wage Campaign, UNISON and Queen Mary College, University of London, September 2001.

8 Mohan, *A National Health Service?* p. 181. In March 2003, the government agreed a new best practice code committing private contractors to pay and conditions for new workers no less favourable than the terms of workers transferred from the public sector. But the code only applies to the local government sector, not to the NHS.

9 On cleaning see the results of a survey reported in the *Guardian* on 10 April 2001, under the heading 'Filthiest NHS hospitals cleaned by private contractors'.

10 According to studies reported by June Carlow in 'Losing their trolley', *Observer*, 11 March 2001. The Department of Health estimated that food rejected by patients cost the NHS £45 million a year (*Guardian*, 13 November 2000).

11 Webster, *The NHS*, p. 158.

12 John Carvel, 'NHS dental pledge after big swing to private care', *Guardian*, 6 January 2003.

13 For a moderate example of the private health care industry's thinking see Health Policy Consensus Group, *Step by Step Reform*, Civitas, London, February 2003.

14 Laing and Buisson, *Health Care Market Review 2003–2004*, London 2003, p. 208.

15 No reliable evidence exists linking the level of fees to the quality of care, and extremes of bad care have been found in care homes charging very high fees. But given that low fees tend to imply fewer staff and/or staff with with lower qualifications, it is widely felt to be better to pay more if you can afford it. See T. Fahey *et al.*, 'Quality of care for elderly residents in nursing homes and elderly people living at home: controlled observational study', *British Medical Journal*, Vol. 326, 2003, p. 580; and S. Jacobs and K. Rummery, 'Nursing homes in England and Wales and their capacity to provide rehabilitation and intermediate care', *Social Policy and Administration* 36:7, 2002, pp. 735–52. A survey of relevant literature is in the PhD thesis of Susan Kerrison, University College London, forthcoming.

16 Declan Gaffney, Allyson Pollock, David Price and Jean Shaoul, 'NHS capital expenditure and the private finance initiative – expansion or contraction?' *British Medical Journal*, Vol. 319, 1999, p. 48.

17 Webster, *The NHS*, p. 151.
18 See e.g. Peter West, *Understanding the National Health Service Reforms*, Open University Press, Buckingham and Philadelphia, 1997.
19 Gaffney *et al.*, 'NHS capital expenditure', p. 48; Office of Health Economics, *Compendium of Health Statistics 2002*, London 2002, Figure 3.10.
20 J. Wilman, 'Patronage determines who serves at the top', *Financial Times*, 14 September 1993.
21 Quoted in Health Policy Network, *In Practice: The NHS Market*, NHSCA, London 1995, p. 13.
22 The figure of 55 per cent relates to unrestricted principals. See Department of Health Statistical Bulletin, *Statistics for Medical Practitioners in England: 1987–1997*.
23 Laing and Buisson, *Health Care Market Review 2003–2004*, p. 79.
24 The quotation is from Julian Tudor Hart, *Feasible Socialism: The National Health Service, Past, Present and Future*, Socialist Health Association, London 1994, p. 27.
25 Derived from *Hansard*, 24 June 1997, part 4, column 667.
26 Increases in costs between the Outline Business Cases and the 1999 costs of fourteen 'first wave' PFI hospitals ranged from 9 per cent for South Bucks to 229 per cent for Wellhouse. The increase was over 50 per cent in half of the hospitals concerned (see Declan Gaffney and Allyson Pollock, 'Pump-priming the PFI: why are privately financed hospital schemes being subsidised?', *Public Money and Management*, January–March 1999, p. 57). For the unsustainable planned bed reductions see Matthew Dunnigan and Allyson Pollock, 'Downsizing of acute inpatient beds associated with the private finance initiative: Scotland's case study', *British Medical Journal*, Vol. 326, 2003, pp. 905–11; and Pollock *et al.*, 'Planning the "new" NHS: downsizing for the 21st century'.
27 S. Pearson, 'Facilities management and outsourcing in the NHS', *British Journal of Health Care Management*, 2/8, 1996, pp. 420–2.
28 Mohan, *A National Health Service?* p. 216.
29 National Audit Office, *Handling Clinical Negligence Claims in England*, HC 403, 2000–01. Claims take a long time to be settled – on average five and a half years for the less serious cases, i.e. those not involving brain damage. For this reason the relevant indices of the cost to the NHS are taken to be the net present value of the predicted final cost of outstanding claims,

and the estimated net present value of the cost of claims not yet made for incidents that have, however, already occurred. The average value of settlements in cases not involving cerebral damage was £87,000, of which one-third was accounted for by legal costs. In 44 per cent of such cases legal costs exceeded the value of the awards made.

30 *Health Service Journal*, 11 December 2003, p. 5.

31 Wanless, *Securing Our Future Health:Taking a Long-term View*, Final Report, p. 83.

32 Guidance letter EL (97) 39, 3 September 1997, paragraph 17.

33 NHS Reform and Health Care Professions Act, 2002.

34 *Delivering the NHS Plan: next steps on investment, next steps on reform*, The Stationery Office, London 2002, p. 16.

35 See e.g. European Commission Directorate General for Regional Policy, 'European Commission – Guidelines for successful public–private partnerships', March 2003.

36 Dunnigan and Pollock, 'Downsizing of acute inpatient beds'.

37 Derek Wanless, *Securing Our Future Health:Taking a Long-term View*, Interim Report, HM Treasury, 2000, pp. 65–8.

38 Department of Health, *Shaping the Future NHS: Long Term Planning for Hospitals and Related Services*, 2000 (the national beds inquiry report). The report examined three 'scenarios'. The 'maintaining trends' and 'acute bed focused' scenarios both called for an *increase* in bed numbers in the short term. The 'care closer to home' scenario allowed for some further decline in bed numbers after 2004, on the basis of some very strong assumptions about increased hospital throughput and 'provided there was a sufficient build-up of community health and social services and intermediate care facilities'.

39 Gaffney and Pollock, 'Pump-priming the PFI', pp. 59–60.

40 Pollock *et al.*, 'Planning the "new" NHS', Tables 1 and 5.

41 See Gaffney *et al.*, 'PFI in the NHS – is there an economic case?', p. 118.

42 See Ibid., pp. 118–19, and, for numerous examples, Allyson M. Pollock, Jean Shaoul, David Rowland and Stewart Player, *Public Services and the Private Sector: a response to the IPPR*, a Catalyst Working Paper, London, November 2001.

43 *Guardian*, 8 February 2002.

44 Allyson M. Pollock, Stewart Player and Sylvia Godden, "How private finance is moving primary care into corporate ownership' , *British Medical*

Journal, Vol. 322, 2001, pp. 960–3, and 'Out of Site', *Guardian*, Society section, 27 February 2002.

45   Pollock *et al.*, *Public Services and the Private Sector*, pp. 41–9.

46   Padma Mallampally and Zbigniev Zimny, 'Foreign direct investment in services', in Yair Aharoni and Lilach Nachum (eds), *Globalisation of Services: some implications for theory and practice*, Routledge, London 2000, pp. 35–6.

47   Karen Stocker, Howard Waitzkin and Celia Iriart, 'The exportation of managed care to Latin America', *New England Journal of Medicine*, 340/14, 1999, pp. 1131–6.

48   David Price, Allyson Pollock and Jean Shaoul, 'How the WTO is shaping domestic policies in health care', *Lancet*, Vol. 354, 1999, pp. 1889–92; and A. M. Pollock and D. Price, 'The public health implications of world trade negotiations on the general agreement on trade in services and public services', *Lancet*, Vol. 362, 2003, pp. 1072–5.

49   *Guardian*, 17 April 2002.

50   *The NHS Plan: a plan for investment and reform*, Cm. 4818-I, The Stationery Office, 2000.

51   See, for example, 'Private sector lobbies for more NHS contracts', *Guardian*, 4 April 2003. Other targets of the private sector included hospital radiology and pathology services.

52   Colin Leys, 'Is consumerism a problem for the NHS?' *Renewal*, 11/2, 2003, pp. 20–8.

53   *The NHS Plan*, p. 96.

54   Department of Health/Independent Healthcare Association, *For the Benefit of Patients: a concordat with the private and voluntary health care provider sector*, Department of Health, 2000.

55   For a partial account of this story see the *Guardian*, 28 July 2000.

56   Department of Health, *Shaping the Future NHS*, p. 13.

57   John Carvel, 'Reid to drop deal with private hospitals', *Guardian*, 6 April 2004.

58   The first 21 DTCs, and their owners, were announced in September 2003 (*Guardian*, 12 September 2003).

59   *Guardian*, 13 January 2004.

60   John Carvel, 'Ministers axe frontrunner in privatised fast-track surgery project', *Guardian*, 6 April 2004.

61   John Carvel, 'Blair puts NHS out to tender', *Guardian*, 14 May 2003.

62   See the supporting documents in Dr Evan Harris, 'Flagship government

private health scheme exposed as rigged and a threat to patient care', Liberal Democrat Briefing Paper, 5 September 2003.

63 *Health Service Journal*, 18 December 2003, p. 7.

64 *Guardian*, 12 September 2003.

65 *Guardian*, 11 September 2003.

66 Health and Social Care Act, 2003.

67 Ian McCartney, 'Keep your nerve; this is the rebirth of popular socialism', *Guardian*, 2 December 2002.

68 *Guardian*, 7 April 2004. The Office of National Statistics took the view that foundation trusts would be privately, not publicly, controlled, because of the lack of public checks on their boards of directors: see ONS, *National Accounts Sector Classifications of NHS Foundation Trusts and NHS Trusts: PSSC decision case 2002/22*, 2 July 2003.

69 Department of Health Response to the Health Select Committee Report on Foundation Trusts, July 2003.

70 London Health Link Discussion Document, August 2003.

71 See e.g. J. G. Williams and R. Y. Mann, 'Hospital episode statistics', *Clinical Medicine*, 2/1, January/February 2002, pp. 34–7.

72 See Richard Cookson, David McDaid and Alan Maynard, 'Wrong SIGN, NICE Mess', *British Medical Journal*, Vol. 323, 2001, pp. 743–5.

73 Patricia Day and Rudolf Klein, 'Who Nose Best?', *Health Service Journal*, 4 April 2000, pp. 26–9.

74 *Delivering the NHS Plan*, p. 38.

4 HOSPITALS

1 It is impossible nowadays to say how many hospitals are included in the NHS because since 1992 hospitals have been administered by trusts and each trust can encompass several hospitals. The last hospital figures available are for 1991.

2 See, for example, G. Fairfield, D. J. Hunter, D. Mechanic, F. Rosleff, 'Managed care: origins, principles and evolution', *British Medical Journal*, Vol. 314, 1997, p. 1823-6; M. Terris, 'Lean and mean: the quality of care in the era of managed care', *Journal of Public Health Policy*, Vol. 19, 1998, pp. 5-14. R. J. Glasser, 'The doctor is not in: on the managed failure of managed medical care', *Harper's Magazine*, March 1998, pp. 35-41.

3   Webster, *The Health Services Since the War*, Vol. I, p. 121. Only 250 hospitals were 'disclaimed' (i.e. not nationalised). These were mainly nursing homes, institutions run by religious orders, and profit-making facilities.

4   Ibid., p. 261.

5   Ibid., p. 262.

6   *Report of the Committee of Enquiry into the Cost of the National Health Services*, (The Guillebaud Report), Cmd. 9663, 1956, p. 132.

7   Ibid., p. 83.

8   John Mohan, *Planning, Markets and Hospitals*, Routledge, London 2002, Chapter 2.

9   Henry Miller, *Medicine and Society*, Oxford University Press, London 1973, p. 50.

10 The Guillebaud Report, p. 72.

11 J. S. Ross, *The National Health Service in Great Britain*, Oxford University Press, London 1952, p. 152.

12 A new reward system, the Clinical Excellence Award Scheme, was introduced in 2003. The scheme sets out 12 award levels ranging from £2,617 at level 1 to £67,097 at level 12. Lower-value awards up to £31,404 will be made by local committees; higher awards will be made by a new national advisory committee. The final salary quoted is for whole-time hospital consultants and excludes discretionary points (which are subsumed in excellence awards) and supplementary payments.

13 Webster, *The Health Services Since the War*, Vol. I, p. 315.

14 A few specialist hospitals such as the Hammersmith Hospital were given the special status of 'special health authority'. However the name 'special health authority' itself indicates that this was a government committed to ensuring that all hospitals planned their services on behalf of geographic populations on the basis of need, not on the basis of any vested or professional interest of their own.

15 House of Commons, *Select Committee on Public Accounts. Twenty Eighth Report*. Session 1998–99.

16 Health Services Act 1976. Although 1,000 paybeds were revoked within 6 months, this still left 3,500 in service. Within a year, the policy of phasing out the remainder at six-monthly intervals had virtually ground to a halt. By the time Labour lost office there were still 2,800 in operation. See Joan Higgins, *The Business of Medicine*, Macmillan, London 1988.

17 Quoted in Mohan, *A National Health Service?*, p. 55.

18 Nicholas Mays, 'Geographical resource allocation in the English National Health Service, 1971–1994: the tension between normative and empirical approaches', *International Journal of Epidemiology*, Vol. 24, 1995, pp. S96–S108.

19 Simon Heffer, *The Life of Enoch Powell*, Weidenfeld & Nicolson, London 1998, p. 290.

20 Ibid., p. 307.

21 Steven Pinch, 'Planning, Markets and Hospitals', *Area*, Vol. 35, 2003, p. 329.

22 Anthony Harrison and Sally Prentice, *Acute Futures*, King's Fund, London 1996, p. 15.

23 Ministry of Health, *NHS Hospital Plan 1962*, Cmnd 1604, London 1962, p. 13.

24 Ibid.

25 Simon Heffer, *The Life of Enoch Powell*, p. 675.

26 Gaffney *et al.*, 'NHS capital expenditure and the private finance initiative', p. 48–51.

27 European Observatory on Health Care Systems, *Health Care Systems in Transition: United Kingdom*, London 1999, p. 63.

28 H. Karcher *et al.*, 'Hospital closures', *British Medical Journal*, Vol. 309, 1994, pp. 973–7.

29 Allyson Pollock *et al.*, 'What happens when the private sector plans hospital services for the NHS? Three case studies under the private finance initiative', *British Medical Journal*, Vol. 314, 1997, p. 1266–71.

30 Department of Health, *Shaping the Future NHS*.

31 Martin McKee and Judith Healy, *Hospitals in a Changing Europe*, Open University Press, Buckingham 2002, p. 6.

32 Matthew Dunnigan and Allyson Pollock, 'Downsizing of acute inpatient beds associated with private finance initiative: Scotland's case study', *British Medical Journal*, Vol. 326, 2003, pp. 905–11.

33 Ibid.

34 Pollock, *et al.*, 'Deficits before Patients'.

35 District Auditor to the Worcestershire Acute Hospitals NHS Trust, *Annual Audit Letter (Audit 2001–2002)*, 26 November 2002.

36 Matthew Dunnigan, *The Downsized Hospital Hypothesis: Value for Money?* NHSCA, Glasgow 2002, pp. 112–19.

37 Ibid.

38 Personal correspondence, letter from Douglas Watt to Malcolm Chisholm, 30 September 2003.

39 Ibid.

40 Dunnigan, *The Downsized Hospital Hypothesis*, pp. 112–19.

41 Ibid.

42 Charles Webster, *The Health Services Since the War*, Vol. II, HMSO, London 1996, p. 767.

43 Richard Crossman, *The Diaries of a Cabinet Minister*, Vol. 3, 1968–1970, Cambridge University Press, London 1977, p. 569.

44 N.W. Chaplin (ed.), *Health Care in the United Kingdom*, Kluwer Medical, London 1982, p. 267.

45 Department of Health and Social Security, *Sharing resources for England. Report of the Resource Allocation Working Party*, London 1976.

46 Mays, 'Geographical resource allocation in the English National Health Service, 1971–1994', pp. 96–102.

47 Chaplin, *Health Care in the United Kingdom*, p. 267

48 Royal Commission on the NHS, *Report of the Royal Commission on the NHS*, Cmnd. 7615, London 1979, p. 348. The idea had first been proposed in 1956.

49 Ibid., p. E.2.2

50 Ibid., p. 350.

51 Department of Health and Social Security, *A Guide for the NHS*, London 1987, p. 3.

52 *Report of the NHS Management Inquiry* (The Griffiths Report), October 1983, pp. 10–11.

53 Higgins, *The Business of Medicine*.

54 McKee and Healy, *Hospitals in a Changing Europe*. And see Alexander Preker and April Harding (eds), *Innovations in Health Service Delivery*, World Bank, Washington 2003.

55 Department of Health and Social Security, *Working for Patients Working Paper 9: capital charges*, London 1989.

56 Mohan, *A National Health Service?* p. 97.

57 Tomlinson quoted in ibid., p. 97.

58 Duncan Nichol, former NHS chief executive, quoted in ibid., p. 13.

59 Paula Mistry, *Rationalising Acute Care Services*, Radcliffe, Oxford 1997, p. 11. By 1999 NHS trusts in Wales had been reduced from 29 to 16 (House of Commons, *Hansard Written Answers*, 24 April 2001, part 9),

Scottish trusts were cut from 47 to 28 (National Audit Office, *NHS (Scotland) Summarised Accounts, 2000*), and NHS trusts in England were cut from 420 to 248 (2003 data only, Department of Health, *Departmental Report 2003*, London 2003). Thus after 1996 total trust numbers in Great Britain fell from 496 to 292, a reduction of 41 per cent.

60 McKee and Healy, *Hospitals in a Changing Europe*, p. 6.

61 Secretary of State for Health, *Working for Patients*, Cm. 555, London 1989.

62 DHSS, *Health Services Development. Health Services Act 1980: private practice in health service hospitals and control of private hospitals developments. Amenity beds*, HC(80)10, London 1980. See also Higgins, *The Business of Medicine*, p. 85. The latest revised code was published by the Department of Health in 2003: Department of Health, *A Code of Conduct for Private Practice: recommended standards for NHS consultants*, London 2003. Like the 1980 code, it is voluntary.

63 House of Commons Health Committee, *The Role of the Private Sector in the NHS*, HC 308-I, May 2002. The committee concluded (conclusions 1 and 2): 'It remains to be demonstrated that greater use of the capacity of the independent sector poses no direct threat to research in the public sector … [We] think it is imperative that the NHS develops sufficient acute capacity.'

64 Laing and Buisson, *Health Care Market Review 2003–2004*, p. 67.

65 Anthony Browne, 'Scandal of NHS beds auction', *Observer*, 6 January 2002.

66 Laing and Buisson, *Health Care Market Review 2003–2004*, p. 79, citing the Health Select Committee, 1999–2000.

67 John Yates, *Private Eye, Heart and Hip: Surgical consultants, the National Health Service and private medicine*, Churchill Livingstone, Edinburgh 1995.

68 *Guardian*, 24 July 2002.

69 Anthony Browne, 'Cash-strapped NHS hospitals chase private patient "bonanza"', *Observer*, 16 December 2001.

70 McKee and Healy, *Hospitals in a Changing Europe*.

71 Mohan, *A National Health Service?* p. 134.

72 North Durham Acute Hospitals NHS Trust, *New DGH for North Durham: full business case*, Durham 1996.

73 European Commission, *Directive Covering Certain Aspects of the Organisation of Working Time*, 93/104/EC, 23 November 1993.

74 The maximum weekly hours of duty including additional duty hours was agreed between the BMA and Department of Health in 1995

(Department of Health, *The New Deal*, London 1995). The deal specified 56 hours for those on full shifts, 64 hours for those working partial shifts, 72 hours for those in hard-pressed on-call posts, and 83 hours for those in non-hard-pressed on-call posts.

75 Audit Scotland, *Catering for Patients*, Edinburgh, November 2003, p. 16.

76 Matthew Fort, 'Hospital food remains in a critical condition', *Guardian*, 14 November 2001.

77 Health Act 1999, Section 18, Duty of quality.

78 Secretary of State for Health, *Learning from Bristol: the report of the public inquiry into children's heart surgery at the Bristol Royal Infirmary 1984–1995*, Cm 5207 (I-III), London July 2001.

79 Department of Health, *Draft Consultants' Contract*, 2003.

80 Audit Commission, *Waiting List Accuracy*, London, 5 March 2003.

81 Alastair McLellan, 'Milburn secured three stars for PM's trust', *Health Service Journal*, 18 December 2003, pp. 3–4; Alastair McLellan and Helen Mooney, 'Ambulance trust gains star boost', *Health Service Journal*, 8 January 2004, pp. 4–5.

82 Peyvand Khaleghian, *Decentralization and Public Services: the case of immunization*, World Bank, Washington, March 2003.

83 Department of Health, 'Government departments must lead efficiency by example Reid tells select committee', press release, 30 October 2003.

84 Department of Health, *Reforming NHS Financial Flows: introducing payment by results*, London 2002, annex 6.

85 Ibid.; Department of Health, *Implementing the New System of Financial Flows – payment by results: technical guidance 2003/04*, London 2002.

86 House of Commons Health Committee, *The Role of the Private Sector in the NHS*.

87 See e.g. Danish Ministry of Health, Hospital Funding and Casemix, Booklet series on health analyses, Copenhagen 1999; Department of Health, *Reforming NHS financial flows*, annex 2.

88 Karin Lowson, Peter West, Stephen Chaplin, and Jacqueline O'Reilly, *Evaluation of Treating Patients Overseas*, Final Report of the York Health Economics Consortium, York 2002.

89 These extensions of 'patient choice' have been extensively influenced by developments in European Union law concerning the free movement of patients in circumstances where national health systems cause undue delay in treatment.

90 Institute of Directors, *Healthcare in the UK: the need for reform*, IOD, London, 2002.

91 Ian McCartney, 'Keep your nerve: this is the rebirth of popular socialism'.

92 Dr Tim Evans, interview with Colin Leys, 30 July 2000.

5 PRIMARY CARE

1 M. Whitehead, 'Equity issues in the NHS: Who cares about equity in the NHS?' *British Medical Journal*, Vol. 308, 1994, pp. 1284–7.

2 K. Caldwell, C. Francome, J. Lister, *The Envy of the World: the past and future of the National Health Service*, NHS Support Foundation, London 1998, p. 26.

3 Julian Tudor Hart, *A New Kind of Doctor*, Merlin Press, London 1998, p. 42.

4 Ministry of Health, *Interim Report on the Future Provision of Medical and Allied Services (Chair, Dawson of Penn)*, Consultative Council on Medical and Allied Services, cmd 693, London, HMSO, 1920.

5 C. Webster, 'The Battle for the Health Centre', *Health Matters*, 1995, No. 2, p. 5.

6 J. A. Scott, H. A. C. Sturgess, *The National Health Service Act 1946*, Eyre & Spottiswoode Ltd, London 1947.

7 *British Medical Journal*, Vol. II, 1944, supplement, pp. 40–41.

8 H. Eckstein, *The English Health Service*, Cambridge, Mass., Harvard University Press, 1970 (Third reprint), p. 152.

9 British Medical Association, *A General Medical Service for the Nation*, British Medical Association, London, November 1938.

10 Eckstein, *The English Health Service*, p. 61.

11 Webster, *The Health Services Since the War*, Vol. I, p. 355.

12 Webster, *The Health Services Since the War*, Vol. II, p. 12.

13 Ibid., p. 84.

14 Central Health Services Council, *Report of the Committee on General Practice of the Central Health Services Council (Chair, Sir Henry Cohen)*, HMSO, London 1954.

15 Geoffrey Rivett, *From Cradle to Grave: fifty years of the NHS*, The King's Fund, London 1988, p. 89.

16 Ministry of Health, *The General Medical Services*, 1953, pp. 51–69.

17 Webster, *The Health Services Since the War*, Vol. I, p. 352.
18 I. Loudon, J. Horder and C. Webster, *General Practice under the National Health Service 1948–1997*, Clarendon Press, Oxford 1998.
19 Radical Statistics Health Group, *Facing the Figures: what really is happening to the National Health Service*, Radical Statistics, London 1989.
20 Department of Health, *Prescriptions dispensed in the Community – Statistics for 1992 to 2002: England*, July 2003. Prescription charges paid by patients covered only about 15 per cent of the total NHS drugs bill.
21 National Audit Office, *General Practitioner Fundholding in England*, HMSO, London 1994.
22 J. Dixon and H. Glennerster, 'What do we know about fundholding in general practice?' *British Medical Journal*, Vol. 311, 1995, pp. 727–30.
23 J. Dixon, 'Can there be fair funding for fundholding practices?', *British Medical Journal*, Vol. 308, 1994, pp. 772–5.
24 House of Commons, *National Health Service Reform and Health Care Professions Act 2002*, The Stationery Office, London, 2002, http://www.hmso.gov.uk/acts/acts2002/20020017.htm.
25 House of Commons, *The National Health Service (Primary Care Act) 1997*, The Stationery Office, London 1997.
26 Royal College of General Practitioners, 'Profile of UK general practitioners', RCGP information sheets No. 1, November 2001, p. 4.
27 PMS National Evaluation team, 'National Evaluation of First Wave NHS Personal Medical Services Pilots, Summary of Findings', March 2002, http://www.npcrdc.man.ac.uk.
28 Ibid., p. 14.
29 Department of Health, *Statistics for General Medical Practitioners in England: 1990–2000*, Bulletin 2001, Vol. 4.
30 S. Gnani and A. M. Pollock, 'The new GMS contract – a Trojan horse?', *British Journal of General Practice*, 2003:53, pp. 354–5.
31 N. Hairon, 'Healthcall gears up for more business', *Pulse*, 17 June 2002, p. 7.
32 M. Benzeval and K. Judge, 'Access to health care in England: continuing inequalities in the distribution of GPs', *Journal of Public Health Medicine*, 1996, Vol. 18, No. 1, pp. 33–40.
33 Department of Health, *Building on the Best – Choice, Responsiveness and Equity in the NHS*, The Stationery Office, London 2003.
34 NHS Executive, *Information for Health: An information strategy for the modern*

NHS, The Stationery Office, London 1998.

35 P. Shekelle and M. Roland, 'Nurse-led telephone-advice lines', *Lancet*, 1999, Vol. 354, p. 88.

36 J. Munro, J. Nicholl, A. O'Cathain and E. Knowles, 'Impact of NHS Direct on demand for immediate care: observational study', *British Medical Journal*, Vol. 321, 2000, pp. 150–3; M. Chalder, D. Sharp, L. Moore and C. Salisbury, 'Impact of NHS walk-in centres on workload of other local healthcare providers: time series analysis', *British Medical Journal*, Vol. 326, 2003, pp. 532–4.

37 Controller and Auditor General, *NHS Direct in England*, National Audit Office, London 2002.

38 Laing and Buisson, *Laing's Healthcare Market Review 1999–2000*, 2000, pp. 137–45.

39 J. Meikle, 'Supermarket offers in-store flu vaccination', *Guardian*, 1 October 2002, society.guardian.co.uk.

40 D. Batty, 'Private health firm plans supermarket sweep', *Guardian*, 29 April 2003, societyguardian.co.uk.

41 Letter to Lambeth, Southwark, and Lewisham Health Authority, 23 August 1994.

42 A. M. Pollock, S. Player, S. Godden, 'How private finance is moving primary care into corporate ownership', *British Medical Journal*, Vol. 322, 2001, pp. 960–3.

43 Department of Health, *NHS, Primary care, general practice and the NHS Plan*, January 2001; J. Kay, 'Surgeries get a cash lift', *Medeconomics*, April 2002, pp. 35–6.

44 G. Clews, 'Time to face LIFT', *BMA News*, September 2002, pp. 13–14.

45 J. Bailey, C. Glendinning and H. Gould, *Better Buildings for Better Services: innovative developments in primary care*, Radcliffe Medical Press, Oxford 1997.

46 A. M. Pollock, 'Will primary care trusts lead to US-style health care?' *British Medical Journal*, Vol. 322, 2001, pp. 964–7.

47 *The NHS Plan*, The Stationery Office, 2000, p. 77.

48 *Delivering the NHS Plan*, The Stationery Office, 2000, p. 30.

49 Press Association, 'Most GPs will ditch night visits, shows survey', *Guardian*, 2 December 2003, societyguardian.co.uk.

50 A. M. Pollock, S. Godden and S. Player. 'Capital investment in primary care – the funding and ownership of primary care premises,' *Public Money and Management*, October–December 2001, pp. 43–9; A. M. Pollock,

S. Godden and S. Player, 'GPs' surgeries turn a profit', *Public Finance*, 2 December 1999, pp. 26–8; A. M. Pollock, 'The American Way', *Health Service Journal*, 9 April 1998, pp. 28–9.

51 John Carvel and Paul Stephenson, 'The American Dream', *Guardian*, 26 May 2004.

6 LONG-TERM CARE FOR OLDER PEOPLE

1 Sir Stewart Sutherland, *With Respect to Old Age: Long Term Care – Rights and Responsibilities: A Report by the Royal Commission on Long Term Care* (The Sutherland Report), *Research*, Vol. 1, London 1999, pp. 8–10.

2 Maria Evandrou, 'Employment and care, paid and unpaid work: the socio-economic position of informal carers in Britain', in J. Phillips (ed.), *Working Carers: international perspectives on working for older people*, Aldershot 1995; Help the Aged, *Caring in Later Life – Reviewing the role of carers*, London 2001.

3 Laing and Buisson, *Care of Elderly People Market Survey 2003*, London 2003.

4 Ibid., Table 2.1.

5 Ibid.

6 Royal College of Physicians, Royal College of Nursing and the British Geriatric Society, *The Health Care of Older People in Care Homes*, London 2000.

7 Research by the Association of Charity Officers in 2001 found that GPs were charging care homes a 'retainer' of £41 per resident in order to provide services to the home (this was despite the fact that GPs automatically receive an NHS capitation fee for each patient over the age of 75 whether they live in their own homes or are residents in a care home). These costs were recouped from the resident by the home owners. Association of Charity Officers, *Fees Paid to GPs for Services to Residents of Care Accommodation for Older People, 2000–2001*, London 2001.

8 Tony Blair MP, *Hansard*, 14 February 2001, Column 314.

9 Alissa Goodman, Michal Myck and Andrew Shephard, *Sharing in the Nation's Prosperity? Pensioner Poverty in Britain*, Institute for Fiscal Studies, London 2003.

10 P. Thompson, '"I don't feel old": subjective ageing and the search for meaning in later life', *Ageing and Society*, Vol. 12, 1992, p. 27; The

Sutherland Report, *Research*, Vol. I, p. 14.

11   The Report of the Working Group on the Implications of Demographic Change, *The Challenge of Longer Life: Economic burden or social opportunity?*, Catalyst, London 2003, p. 17.

12   *Royal Commission on Population*, London 1949, p. 113: quoted in Robin Means and Randall Smith, *From Poor Law to Community Care – the development of welfare services for elderly people 1939–1971*, Bristol 1998, p. 212.

13   *The Challenge of Longer Life.*

14   Paul Burstow, 'The scandal of long-term care under Labour – A survey of the number of people forced to sell their home to pay for nursing or residential care', Liberal Democrats, London 2001.

15   Aneurin Bevan MP, *Hansard*, Vol. 443, 24 November 1947, Column 1609, quoted in Means and Smith, *From Poor Law to Community Care*, p. 139.

16   Ibid.

17   Laing and Buisson, *Care of Elderly People Market Survey 1985*, London 1985, p. 14.

18   Means and Smith, *From Poor Law to Community Care*, p. 248.

19   Martin Knapp, Brian Hardy and Julien Forder, *Commissioning for Quality: ten years of social care markets in England*, Discussion paper 1600, Personal Social Services Research Unit, Kent 2000, p. 7.

20   Ministry of Health Circular 18/65, London 1965, quoted in Means and Smith, p. 186.

21   Robin Means, 'Lesson from the history of long term care for older people', in Janice Robinson, (ed.), *Towards a New Social Compact for Care in Old Age*, Kings Fund, London 2001, p. 21.

22   Ibid.

23   G. Sumner and R. Smith, *Planning Local Authority Services for the Elderly*, London 1969, p. 25, quoted in Means and Smith, p. 167.

24   Means and Smith, *From Poor Law to Community Care*, p.169.

25   Robin Means, Hazel Morbey and Randall Smith, *From Community Care to Market Care? – the development of welfare services for older people*, Bristol 2002, p. 52.

26   Mark Drakeford, *Privatisation and Social Policy*, Harlow 2000, p. 103.

27   Saul Becker, *Responding to Poverty – The Politics of Cash and Care*, London 1997, p. 122.

28   Alan Walker, 'More ebbs than flows', *Social Service Insight*, 29 March 1986, pp. 16–17.

29   Laing and Buisson, *Care of Elderly People Market Survey 1998*, London 1998, p. 29.

30   Laing and Buisson, *Care of Elderly People Market Survey 2003*, London 2003, pp. 35–6.

31   Becker, *Responding to Poverty*, p. 124.

32   Ibid., p. 123.

33   Laing and Buisson, *Care of Elderly People Market Survey 1994*, London 1994.

34   Laing and Buisson, *Care of Elderly People Market Survey 2003*, London 2003.

35   Gerald Wistow, 'The changing scene in Britain', in Tessa Harding (ed.), *Options for Long Term Care: economic, social and ethical choices*, London 1996, p. 65.

36   Audit Commission, *Making a Reality of Community Care*, London 1986.

37   Sir Roy Griffiths, *Community Care: Agenda for Action*, London 1988.

38   Virginia Bottomley MP, quoted in House of Commons Health Committee, *Third Report – Community Care: Funding from April 1993 Volume II – Minutes of Evidence and Appendices*, London 1993, p. 18.

39   R v. Wandsworth London Borough Council ex parte Beckwith (1996) 1 All ER 129.

40   Accounts Commission, *Dumfries and Galloway Council Externalisation of Residential Homes for Older People*, Scotland 2000.

41   A. Netten, A. Bebbington, R. Darton, J. Forder, K. Miles, *1996 Survey of Care Homes for Elderly People (Final Report)*, Personal Social Services Research Unit Discussion paper 1423/2, Kent 1998.

42   Secretaries of State for Health and Social Security, Wales and Scotland, *Caring for People: Community Care in the Next Decade and Beyond*, London 1989.

43   Becker, *Responding to Poverty*, pp. 134–5.

44   Wistow, 'The changing scene in Britain', p. 63.

45   Ibid., p.64.

46   W. K. Reid, *Failure to Provide Long Term NHS Care for a Brain Damaged Patient: Report of the Health Service Commissioner*, London 1994.

47   Department of Health Circulars HSG[95]8 and LAC [95]50, London 1995.

48   'ACC survey claims £116m loss from budgets', *Community Care Market News*, April 1996.

49 Help the Aged, *Nothing Personal – Rationing Social Care for Older People*, London 2002.

50 Becker, *Responding to Poverty*, p. 144.

51 Local Government Anti-Poverty Unit, *Survey of Charges for Social Care 1993–1995*, London 1995, quoted in Becker, p. 140.

52 Audit Commission, *Charging with Care: How Councils Charge for Home Care*, London 2000.

53 Ibid.

54 Becker, *Responding to Poverty*, p. 141.

55 House of Commons Health Committee, 'Public Expenditure on Health and Social Services', yearly memoranda 1992–2000, London.

56 Becker, *Responding to Poverty*, p. 142.

57 Netten, *et al.*, *1996 Survey of Care Homes*, Table 2.8.

58 Ibid.

59 The Sutherland Report, Executive Summary and Summary of Recommendations, London 1999.

60 Ibid.

61 Chris Deeming, *A Fair Deal for Older People? Public views on the funding of long-term care*, London 2001.

62 Joel Joffe and David Lipsey, 'Note of Dissent', in The Sutherland Report, Main Report, para. 4.

63 Tony Blair MP, *Hansard*, 14 February 2001, Column 314.

64 R v. North and East Devon Health Authority ex parte Coughlan, Court of Appeal 1999.

65 Health Service Ombudsman, *NHS Funding for Long Term Care*, 2nd Report Session 2002–2003 HC 399, London 2003.

66 David Batty, 'Elderly pay for "free" nursing care', *Guardian*, January 28 2002.

67 'Elderly denied free nursing care', BBC News, 28 January 2002, www.news.bbc.co.uk.

68 David Batty, 'Move to block unfair care home fees "will not work"', *Guardian*, 11 March 2002.

69 John Hutton MP, *Hansard*, 3 April 2000, Column 789.

70 Laing and Buisson, *Care of Elderly People Market Survey 1998*, London 1998, p. 29.

71 Paul Boateng, quoted in 'Partnerships must be way forward', *Community Care Market News*, May 1998.

72 Department of Health, *Capital Investment Strategy*, London 1999.

73 'Additional £100m Winter Pressures Money in PSS Settlement for 2001–2002', *Community Care Market News*, December 2000/January 2001.

74 PricewaterhouseCoopers, *Survey of Personal Social Services Assets, Strategies and Management – A Research Report*, London 2000; Department of Health, *Community Care Statistics 2002*, London 2002.

75 Department of Health, *A Guide to Contracting for Intermediate Care Services*, London 2001.

76 Laing and Buisson, *Care of Elderly People Market Survey 2002*, London 2002.

77 Charlene Harrington, David Zimmerman, Sarita L. Karon, James Robinson, and Patricia Beutel, 'Nursing home staffing and its relationship to deficiencies', *Journal of Gerontology: Social Sciences*, Vol. 55B, 2000, pp. 5278–87.

78 Jeremy Kendall, 'Of knights, knaves and merchants: the case of residential care for older people in England in the late 1990s', *Social Policy and Administration*, Vol. 35, No. 4, September 2001, pp. 360–75.

79 See http://www.alchemypartners.co.uk.

80 S. Player and A. Pollock, 'Long term care from public responsibility to private good', *Critical Social Policy*, Vol. 21, May 2001.

81 Jacquetta Williams, Ann Netten, Brian Hardy, Tihana Matosevic and Patricia Ware, *Care Home Closures: the provider perspective*, Personal Social Services Research Unit Discussion paper 1753/2, Kent 2002.

82 'Watchdog urged for care homes', the charity Counsel and Care, which campaigns for better care for older people, quoted in the *Guardian*, 5 April 2000.

83 Williams *et al.*, *Care Home Closures*, p. 40.

84 Laing and Buisson, *Care of Elderly People Market Survey 2003*, London 2003, Table 5.1, p. 90.

85 John Hutton MP, *Hansard*, 19 July 2000, Column 218W.

86 Professor David Jolley, 'A report to the High Court of Justice Queen's bench division, Administrative Court, case references: CO/5147/2002 and CO/2278/2002, February 2003.

87 National Audit Office, *Ensuring the Effective Discharge of Older Patients from NHS Acute Hospitals*, HC 392 Session 2002–2003, London 2003.

88 David Rowland and Allyson Pollock, 'Choice and responsiveness for older

people in the "patient centred" NHS', *British Medical Journal*, Vol. 328, 2003, p. 4.

89 Social and Health Care Workforce Group, *Independent Sector Workforce Survey 2001 Provisional Report*, Employers Organisation, London 2002; Local Government Management Board, *Independent Sector Workforce Survey 1996 – Residential and nursing homes in Great Britain*, London 1997

90 Adelina Comas-Herrera, Tihana Matosevic and Jeremy Kendall, 'The social care workforce', in Melanie Henwood (ed.), *Future Imperfect*, London 2001, p. 208.

91 Ibid., p. 209; Social and Health Care Workforce Group, *Independent Sector Workforce Survey 2001 Provisional Report*.

92 Ginny Jenkins, Zee Asif, Gerry Bennett, *Listening Is Not Enough*, Action on Elder Abuse, London 2000.

93 Ginny Jenkins, quoted in David Brindle, 'Study uncovers care home abuse', *Guardian*, 7 February 2000.

94 C. Harrington, D. Zimmerman, S. Karon, J. Robinson and P. Beutel, 'Nursing home staffing and its relationship to deficiencies', *Journal of Gerontology*, 2000; Vol. 55, pp, 278–87; C. Harrington, H. Carrillo, S. Thollaug and P. Summers, *Nursing Facilities, Staffing, Residents and Facility Deficiencies 1993–99. Report for the Health Care Financing Administration*, San Francisco, University of California 2000, http://www.hcfa.gov/medicaid/nursingfac/nursfac99.pdf.

95 Department of Health, *Fit for the Future? National Required Standards for Residential and Nursing Homes for Older People*, London 1999, p. 70.

96 Ibid.

97 John Carvel, 'Milburn retreats on care home standards', *Guardian*, 20 August 2002.

98 'The 15 most powerful people in health', and 'The 15 most powerful people in social care', *Guardian*, 14 November 2000.

99 'The 15 most powerful people in social care'.

100 Kendra Inman, 'Cut to the bone', *Guardian*, 5 July 2000.

101 *Community Care Market News*, March 2001, p. 204; 'Profile of Chai Patel' *Guardian*, 25 September 2002.

102 Jay Rayner, 'A home unfit for heroes', *Observer*, 9 June 2002.

103 Jo Revill, 'Blair adviser quits in nursing home scandal', *Observer*, 22 September 2002.

104 'Lynde House Report', *Richmond and Twickenham Times*, 29 August 2002.

105 www.englishcare.org.
106 'Care home owners ready for action if calls for fee increases go ignored', *Community Care Market News*, May 2003.
107 'Protest on fee levels', *Community Care Market News*, December 2000/ January 2001.
108 'Scottish Care and COSLA enter into negotiations to end fees row', *Community Care Market News*, August/September 2001; 'COSLA agrees to contribute to fee increases', *Community Care Market News*, March 2002.
109 'Provider pressure forces up fee rates', *Community Care Market News*, June 2002.
110 'Care homes warned on cartels', *Community Care Market News*, November 2003, p. 1.
111 Melanie McFadyean and David Rowland, *Selling off the Twilight Years: The transfer of Birmingham's homes for older people*, London 2002.
112 John Carvel, 'Pensioner, 102, leads eviction protest to No. 10', *Guardian*, 19 March 2002.
113 R (Heather) v. Leonard Cheshire Foundation [2001] EWHC Admin 429. In his judgement Lord Justice Stanley Burton commented on the difference between state-owned and private-owned care homes and their different responsibilities when confronted by financial difficulties. At paragraph 71 he stated: 'it should be borne in mind that non-governmental bodies often differ from governmental authorities in relation to their financial resources. Whereas private bodies must nearly always balance their income and expenditure, at least over the medium term, and have limited assets and income, governmental bodies may have access to tax revenues. … A purely private body is, within legal constraints, generally entitled to act in its own economic interests; it will often be compelled to act in those interests'.
114 William Laing, *Disparities Between Market Rates and State Funding of Residential Care*, Joseph Rowntree, York 1998.
115 Laing and Buisson, *Care of Elderly People Market Survey 2002*, London 2002, p.49

7 OVERCOMING OPPOSITION

1 Patrick Wintour and Kevin Maguire, 'Private contractors cut jobs to save cash', *Guardian*, 8 March 2002

2   'Dudley strikes a blow against PFI', *Public Finance Magazine*, 27 April 2001.

3   HM Treasury, *PFI: Meeting the Investment Challenge*, The Stationery Office, London July 203, Chapter 6, Employee Protection.

4   Jo-Ann Mulligan, 'What do the public think?' in John Appleby and Anthony Harrison (eds), *Health Care UK: The King's Fund Review of Health Policy*, Winter 2000, The King's Fund, London 2000, p. 14.

5   See Allyson M. Pollock, M. Dunnigan, D. Gaffney, A. MacFarlane and F. A. Majeed, 'What happens when the private sector plans hospital services for the NHS: three case studies under the private finance initiative', *British Medical Journal*, Vol. 314, 1997, pp. 1266–71.

6   Lynn Eaton, 'Happy Clappy', *Health Service Journal*, 14 February 2002, pp. 9–10.

7   Personal communication to the author.

8   *The NHS Plan*.

9   Anthony Browne, 'Why the NHS is bad for us', *Observer*, 7 October 2001.

10 Conrad F. Meier, 'Health care in England: Not your cup of tea: Introduction', *Health Care News*, 1 September 2001.

11 Elizabeth Warren, Teresa Sullivan, Melissa Jacoby, 'Medical Problems and Bankruptcy Filings', *Norton's Bankruptcy Adviser*, May 2000.

12 'HMOs the new nasties', *Economist*, 9 July 1998.

13 Personal communication to the author.

14 Tash Shifrin, 'Good Vibrations?' *Health Service Journal*, 27 June 2002, p. 15; Department of Health, *Delivering the NHS Plan*, p. 26.

15 World Health Organisation, *World Health Report 2000. Health systems: improving performance*, Geneva 2000.

16 Alan Williams, 'Science or marketing at WHO?' *Health Economics*, Vol. 10, Issue 2, March 2001, pp. 93–100.

17 Anna Dixon and Elias Mossialos, 'Social insurance: not much to write home about?, *Health Service Journal*, 24 January 2002, pp. 24–6.

18 Paul Webster, 'NHS in crisis? Patients in France also wait on Trolleys', *Observer*, 7 December 2003.

19 Labour Research press release, 2 June 2002.

20 Bobbie Jacobson, Jenny Mindell, Martin McKee, 'Hospital mortality league tables', *British Medical Journal*, Vol. 326, 2003, pp. 777–8.

21 H Goldstein, D. J. Spiegelhalter, 'League Tables and their limitations: statistical issues in comparisons of institutional performance,' *Journal of the Royal Statistical Society*, Series A, Vol. 159, 1996, pp. 385–443.

22 Patrick Butler, 'Trust Chief quits following waiting list scandal,' *Guardian*, 14 March 2001.

23 For one example among many see the case of Dr Geeta Nargund who was suspended for fifteen months after protesting about staff shortages and the promotion of a doctor involved in an embryo mix-up at St George's Hospital in Tooting (Rebecca Allison, 'Suspended consultant reinstated', *Guardian*, 23 January 2004).

24 Judy Jones, 'The secret life of the NHS', *British Medical Journal*, Vol. 320, 2000, pp. 1457–9.

25 Sheldon Rampton and John Stauber, 'Research Funding, Conflicts of Interest and the "Meta-Methodology" of Public Relations', *Public Health Reports*, Vol. 17, July–August 2002, pp. 331–9.

26 Ibid.; for more details on the Olivieri case see the Canadian Association of University Teachers website: www.caut.ca.

27 Richard Smith, 'PFI: Perfidious Financial Idiocy', *British Medical Journal*, Vol. 319, 1999, pp. 2–3.

28 Sarah Boseley, 'BMA out of touch with doctors, says Blair', *Guardian*, 8 July 1999.

29 Judy Jones, 'The private finance initiative: spinning out the defence', *British Medical Journal*, Vol. 320, 2000, pp 1460–1.

30 Reeves left the Department of Health to head the Accountancy Foundation Review Board before going on to join the private sector when the Review Board folded in September 2003 (Accountancy Foundation 'Press Notice', 5 September 2003).

31 Jones, 'The private finance initiative'. Jones reported 'rumours' that the article had been commissioned by the Department from outside authors and not submitted to the *British Medical Journal* for many months because it was seen as a largely ad hominem attack on the authors of the original *British Medical Journal* articles.

32 P. Coates, 'Don't Shoot the Messenger', *Public Finance*, 25 August 2000, pp. 16–19.

33 House of Commons Health Committee, *Minutes of Evidence taken before the Health Committee: Public Expenditure and the National Plan*, 2 November 2000, The Stationery Office, London, HC 957-i, Questions 169–79.

34 Department of Health, 'Bed numbers and NBI Compliance in Capital Development Schemes', unpublished paper, 22 September 2000.

35 Matthew Dunnigan and Allyson Pollock, 'Downsizing of acute inpatient

beds associated with private finance initiative: Scotland's case study', pp. 905–8.

36 G. Harris, 'New PFI hospital branded a failure', *The Times*, 26 April 2003.

37 R. Dinwoodie and A. McDermid, 'New study condemns Labour's hospital policy', *Glasgow Herald*, 25 April 2003.

38 Reporting Scotland, BBC1, 25 April 2003; R. Dinwoodie, 'Litany of faults cited as PFI row rages on', *Glasgow Herald*, 26 April 2003.

39 Tara Womersley, 'ERI "stumbles" at first winter hurdle', *Scotsman*, 15 January 2004; *Edinburgh Evening News*, 'Go-ahead for hospital probe', 16 January 2004.

40 Richard G. A. Feachem, Neelam K. Sekhri, Karen L. White, Jennifer Dixon, Donald M. Berwick, and Alain C. Enthoven, 'Getting more for their dollar: a comparison of the NHS with California's Kaiser Permanente', *British Medical Journal*, Vol. 324, 2002, p. 135–43.

41 To view these emails see *Rapid Responses* on the *British Medical Journal* website, www.bmj.com.

42 The authors' purported adjustments did not take into account the ways in which the populations of patients served by Kaiser Permanente and the NHS are fundamentally different. Kaiser Permanente's patients are mainly employed, and significantly younger; Kaiser Permanente has barely half the proportion of people over 75 that the NHS looks after. They are also significantly less socially deprived and so are healthier. Feachem and his co-authors attempted to adjust for these factors but failed to do so adequately. On top of this they inflated the NHS's costs by about 40 per cent through an elementary statistical mistake; and they ignored the cost of vital services including training and research which the NHS provides and Kaiser Permanente does not – precisely because the NHS is an integrated and hence more efficient system than the one in which Kaiser Permanente operates; see A. Talbot-Smith, S. Gnani, A. M. Pollock and D. Pereira Gray, 'Questioning the claims from the Kaiser', *British Medical Journal of Practice*, Vol. 54, 2004, pp. 415–21.

43 A selection of emails was printed later, with a sadly superficial commentary. 'Letters: Getting more for their dollar: Kaiser vs the NHS', *British Medical Journal*, Vol. 324, 2002, pp. 1332–5.

44 Chris Ham, Nick York, Steve Sutch, and Rob Shaw, 'Hospital bed utilisation in the NHS, Kaiser Permanente, and the US Medicare programme: analysis of routine data', *British Medical Journal*, Vol. 327, 2003,

pp. 1257–60; Donald Light and M. Dixon, 'Making the NHS more like Kaiser Permanente', *British Medical Journal*, Vol. 328, 2004, pp. 763–75.

45 David S. David, 'RE: Lessons for the NHS from Kaiser Permanente, hospital bed utilization', Letter to the editor, *British Medical Journal*, 16 December 2003; www.bmj.com.

46 House of Commons Health Committee, *The Role of the Private Sector in the NHS*, Stationery Office, London 2002, Vol. I.

47 *The Role of the Private Sector*, Vol. II, Minutes of Evidence, Q. 396.

48 Matthew Norman, 'Diary', *Guardian*, 22 May 2002; 'Woman in the eye: Julia Drown', *Private Eye*, No. 1055, 31 May–13 June 2002.

49 Roy Hattersley, 'The perils of plain speaking', *Guardian*, 25 May 2002; Dr Richard Taylor MP, Letter to the Editor, *Guardian*, 25 May 2002.

50 John Carvel, 'PFI critic demands retraction after "sloppy research" accusation by MPs', *Guardian*, 1 June 2002.

8 THE EMERGING HEALTH CARE MARKET

1 Kable Ltd, 'Health ICT market profile to 2008', London 2003.

2 Tony Blair, 'Progressive governance', *Progressive Politics*, January 2003, Vol. 2/1, p. 9.

3 John Reid MP, *Minutes of Evidence for Thursday 30 October 2003: Public Expenditure 2003, House of Commons Health Committee*, The Stationery Office, London, HC 1109-ii, Question 224.

4 Steffie Woolhandler, Terry Campbell and David Himmelstein, 'Costs of health care administration in the United States and Canada', *New England Journal of Medicine*, Vol. 349, 21 August 2003, pp. 768–75.

5 *Guardian*, 7 April 2004; see also Rudolph Klein, 'The first wave of the NHS foundation trusts', *British Medical Journal*, Vol. 328, 2004, p. 1332.

INDEX

Mistry, Paula 104–5
mixed economy 164
    of health care 11–12, 62–78, 118,
    133–45, 168
    of primary care 153
Montague, Adrian 5–6
Morecambe NHS Trust 11–12
mortality data 100, 117
motor neurone disease 87
Moyes, Bill 8, 218
Mulgan, Geoff 3
multinational corporations 9–10, 34
    health care companies 123
multiple sclerosis 22

National Assistance Act (1948) 160,
    161, 169
national beds inquiry 55, 67, 95
NHS Consultants' Association 8
NHS Management Enquiry (Griffiths)
    101
National Health Services Act (1946)
    160–61
National Health Service
    budgets 22
    clinical care 103
    and Community Care Act 8, 134,
        168
    consultants 68
    denigrating its achievement
        195–7
    dentistry 39, 63
    direct 144–5
    district planning teams 26
    Executive Regional Offices 45
    expenditure 217
    founding principles 78

hospital
    building projects 53
    trusts, 'failing' 122–3
    and Kaiser Permanente 207–9
    nursing staff 41
    PFI unit 4, 206, 210
    plan 62–3, 71, 122
    privatising of 34–80
    Regional Offices
        'entrepreneurialism' 54
    Scotland 8
    selling out 13–16
    spending distribution 82
    staff 41, 202–4
    surgeons 68
    teaching hospitals 109
    walk-in centres 144–5
National Health Service (Primary
    Care) Act (1997) 138
National Health Service, A (1944)
    (White Paper) 128
National Institute for Clinical
    Excellence (NICE) 76–7
National Insurance 127
National Service Frameworks 63, 76
national tariff 73–5, 119–22, 218–19,
    224
neonatal
    deaths in Bristol 116
    heart surgery 115
    intensive care services 73
    surgeons, medical scandal 76
New Labour 220
    commitments to NHS 66
    and EU 61
    fragmentation of NHS under
        49–62